THE HOT SEX HANDBOOK

Also by Tracey Cox

HOT SEX
HOT RELATIONSHIPS

THE HOT SEX HANDBOOK

TRACEY COX

BANTAM BOOKS
NEW YORK • TORONTO • LONDON • SYDNEY • AUCKLAND

THE HOT SEX HANDBOOK
A Bantam Book

PUBLISHING HISTORY
Bantam Australia edition published 2002 (as *A Bit on the Side:
The Hot Sex Handbook*)
Bantam trade paperback edition / August 2005

Published by
Bantam Dell
A Division of Random House, Inc.
New York, New York

Book design by Cheryl Collins Design
Cover design/concept: Cheryl Collins

Library of Congress Catalog Card Number: 2004065575

ISBN 0-553-38347-7

Printed in the United States of America
Published simultaneously in Canada

www.bantamdell.com

BVG 10 9 8 7 6 5 4 3

To those who've already had Hot Sex
but still want more

Contents

....

Introduction

··

Nearly everyone talks about sex. We're always boasting about how *fabulous* so-and-so is in bed and hinting at the real reason why we look so tired at work (nudge, nudge, wink, wink). But it's a rare person who'll confess details or talk specifics. Jane might well confide that Brad gives the best oral sex she's ever had but she doesn't launch into a lick-by-lick analysis of *why*—and I bet you don't ask for one.

That's why we buy sex books—to find out the nitty-gritty details about things we're too embarrassed to ask friends or lovers. Trouble is, few deliver what we really want to know. Sex manuals tend to gloss over the practical bread-and-butter stuff and, instead, talk in generalities—like how women need clitoral stimulation and men's bottoms are a veritable hot spot. Great advice, but if you haven't got the foggiest of what to do with it, useless.

This is where *The Hot Sex Handbook* is different. Instead of assuming you know everything, I've assumed you know nothing and have dished up *all* the gory details in an easy-to-follow, step-by-step format. The only way I could have been more explicit and specific is to be there in the bedroom with you, guiding your hands and whatever else you're using (and, to tell the truth, I'd really rather not).

That's not to say the book *only* deals with the basics. Experienced lovers will get heaps out of *The Hot Sex Handbook* because there are enough advanced tips, tricks, and techniques to keep even Madame Lash happy. But I *do* suggest you don't skip over what might appear to be the "basics." Very often it's the people who *think* they know what they're doing who need educating the most. Sex is a bit like typing. You can get by using two fingers, but you'll never be as good as someone who did the secretarial course and practiced every night. Going back to the grassroots level, even if it's just to check that you're on the right track, isn't a bad idea for all of us. Don't let anyone tell you otherwise: sex skills can be learned and we can *all* improve on them.

I've written the book using everyday language for similar reasons. The correct, technical terms sound terribly authoritative but if *you* don't know that a wet dream is actually called a nocturnal emission, you wouldn't have a clue what I was talking about if I used this term. Sometimes, the words I use aren't even accurate. Most people say *sperm* when they actually mean *semen,* for instance. But, hey, if that's what you call it, that's what I've called it a lot of the time because I want you to relate to what I'm saying.

I'm also guilty of making some broad generalizations about sex. I hope there aren't too many but if you read something that you personally don't agree with, forgive me. If I covered every single individual preference, research finding, exception, and extreme, I'd still be madly typing away at my computer!

I hope you enjoy reading *The Hot Sex Handbook* as much as I enjoyed writing it. Now get to it—shred those sheets!

Wicked Ways to Warm Up

·······································

Anyone can be good in bed. Genital size doesn't matter. Looks don't matter. You don't have to have legs up to your chin or arms like Arnie, drive a sports car, or be rolling in it to be the best lover your partner's ever had. But you do need a good, working knowledge of your subject. Don't let anyone tell you otherwise: sex skills can be learned, we can all improve on them, and I can't think of a better place to start than with foreplay.

It takes the average man two to three

minutes of direct sexual stimulation with a partner to orgasm. It takes the average woman twenty to thirty minutes. You don't need to be Einstein to figure out that if you spend longer on foreplay and master it, you'll need to swap your Little Black Book for a Big Black Briefcase to lug around all your phone numbers. And women aren't the only ones who like foreplay. Even men who can get an erection by inserting a coin in a slot machine can't deny that a good, slow, erotic "tease" dramatically heightens all sexual sensation. Convinced it's imperative you get it right? Thought so! Now, here's some suggestions to improve *your* foreplay finesse.

WHY YOU SHOULD MASTURBATE IN FRONT OF EACH OTHER

Partners can't read minds. So get rid of that "If he/she truly loved me, they'd know what turns me on" stuff right now. Body language can speak volumes and talking to each other is essential, but as the saying goes, a picture is worth a thousand words. Watching each other masturbate, you see firsthand what technique you each use—the pressure and speed, how you speed it up or slow it down on approach to orgasm, how you stimulate yourself (or not) while you're actually having an orgasm, and what you do with your spare hand. All you need to do then is copy each other.

Generally, men are more comfortable masturbating than women are. If your girlfriend's the I'm-game-for-anything type, doing it in front of her may simply be a matter of taking a hold of yourself during foreplay. Chances are, she'll sit back and watch—lots of women are *fascinated*. If she ignores what you're doing, simply say, "I've had fantasies about masturbating in front of you. This feels great." If she still doesn't get the hint and watch add, "This is how I do it when you're not around. Watch." If you want her to imitate your technique, get her to put her hand over yours so she can feel the pressure and rhythm you're using. Ask her to copy you and give lots of positive feedback—"Wow! You're better at it than I am." Uninhibited women can easily apply the same principles.

Your partner's a little shy and so are you?

Talk about it first. Say you watched a show; a friend told you; you read about how watching each other masturbate will improve your sex life immeasurably. Ask if your partner agrees and suggest that the next time you make love, you try it. Don't be concerned if it all seems a bit serious and uncomfortable the first time round. Start by showing one technique you use: come on—that's a mere second or two of embarrassment! And get them to do the same. Later, when you both feel more comfortable, you'll be more confident and relaxed about bringing yourself to an actual orgasm. Masturbating in front of your partner or watching them masturbate has always been up there with the most popular male sex fantasies—and the new breed of sexually liberated females are adding it to *their* list.

DELICIOUS DETOURS

"Happiness isn't a destination; it's a means of traveling." This old saying can be applied to foreplay. Rush through the "traveling" and you might find the destination isn't quite as exciting as you'd expected. Lavish attention on the *whole body* and you can't help but take your time.

Erogenous zones are areas on our bodies that create intense sexual arousal when stimulated. Apart from the obvious bits that we all share (like the penis and the clitoris), each of us has our own secret area that sends frantic *yes! yes!* messages to all the right places. For some, it's being bitten in the small of their neck. Others go crazy when someone strokes their buttocks. But what works for one lover won't necessarily work on the next, so consider each new lover unexplored territory. There are few places on our bodies that we don't like being touched. Why restrict foreplay to the breasts and genitals when the entire body is itching for attention?

- **Take a body tour.** When you get to a new

city, you often take an orientation tour to get your bearings, right? Then what's stopping you from doing the same with your new lover's body? You can go all out here and even use a few props. Make him lie down naked on his stomach and close his eyes—make sure the room you're in is private and warm—then trail a scarf slowly and tantalizingly across his naked bottom and back. Then turn him over and stroke a feather around his penis and scrotum. You can then move on to using your hands, hair, breasts, and mouth on his nipples and genital area, creating different sensations as you search for his ultimate pleasure zones.

- **Try stroking her face,** the back of her neck, her back. Play with her hair, lift it up from her neck and stroke underneath, slide your palms up and down her arms—and this is just while you're watching TV together. Don't even make it to the bedroom.

- **Massage his feet,** kiss his toes, massage his hands, then take each finger into your mouth and suck it, pretending it's his penis.

- **Don't dive straight for his penis during foreplay.** Use long, sensual strokes up his inner thighs until he's *trembling* with desire.
- **Bottoms up!** Both your bottoms are an arousable area. Try massaging them, stroking, even gentle slapping. Don't neglect the perineum (the bit between your genitals and your anus). Press firmly and massage with two fingers, gently stroking along the entire length; use your tongue to do the same.
- **Use your fingers to rub along the outline of his lips,** then insert a finger into his mouth for him to suck. Do the same with your nipples. He can do the same with his penis.
- **Get into neck nibbling.** Do you know anyone who doesn't enjoy having their neck kissed or gently nibbled? (If you do, they're either incredibly ticklish or totally uptight.) It's a sadly ignored area that can produce amazing results.
- **Suck her toes,** slide your tongue into her belly button (try diving on her after a

shower if you're paranoid about "fluff").
Have fun with foreplay! It really doesn't matter if she laughs instead of sighs—she's still complimented that you find *all* of her sexy, not just "the good bits."

> "I met a girl at a bar who looked me straight in the eye then said, 'I want you inside me,' within five minutes of meeting her. This happened at around 9 P.M. and we didn't sleep together until the early hours of the morning, but I was in a state of high excitement from that moment on. That's what I call good foreplay."
> Simon, 29, sales representative

- **Kiss all over his body,** not just on his mouth and genitals.
- **Use your whole body to massage his.** Lie on top of him when he's lying on his back or front, gyrate slowly, and revel in the simple sensation of skin against skin.

And for my next trick . . .

- **Tie him up.** We've all seen it done in the movies. You don't need to pop down to a sex shop and buy one of those leather numbers to slip on (unless you want to, of course) or crack a whip (ditto) to play the dominatrix. But you *do* need a bedpost (or chair) to tie him to, a couple of long scarves (some old stockings or a few of his ties will do), and a nasty smile on your face. Once he's comfortably trussed (don't cut off the circulation, you need the blood flowing for him to get an erection, let alone keep his heart pumping), you can try out a number of erotic scenarios, like . . .

- **Masturbate for him.** Watching you give yourself pleasure will give him a big kick. The effect will be even more spectacular if you masturbate loudly and theatrically while he's tied up and is utterly helpless. If you want to get him *really* worked up, simply leave him tied up and then . . .

- **Blindfold him.** Even a see-through chiffon scarf can increase the sexual tension tenfold. It also makes you less inhibited about what you do to him because he can't see you. Tie the scarf across his eyes, then build the anticipation by withdrawing completely for a few seconds, then caressing him in his favorite places, and a few he's not expecting. This also lets his imagination run wild—you could be a provocative French maid, slave girl . . . you get the picture.

- **Undress each other.** Don't just fling your clothes in a corner and hop into bed naked; let him undress you and vice versa. Stop along the way to lick and caress the body part that's just been exposed.

- **Play the vamp.** Thought the only time you'd use those long, black gloves was on black-tie occasions? Put them on now and start masturbating him. Yes, it does come out in the wash.

- **Make it good enough to eat.** Whipped cream, bananas, and berries aren't just good for fruit salads. Take them out of the kitchen or, better still, stay there and satisfy two appetites at once. Having a feast off each other's bodies is a laugh more than anything else, but even

Whipped cream, ice cream, and chocolate spread . . . they're the three foods 30 percent of women would most like their partners to lick off their body.

if it simply makes sex more fun, it's worth the experiment. Unless you're talking hot and spicy foods, it's safe to smother or insert most foods in and around the genitals for both of you to devour. While you're at it, grab some ice cubes from the freezer, put them into your mouth, then suck his penis.

- **Drop it.** Leave the sisterhood stuff outside the bedroom door. If he fantasizes about you dressing up as a waitress, serving him exactly what he hungers for, he *is* treating you like a sex object—but isn't that the point?

- **Go for the cliché**—most men love it. Invest in some sexy black underwear. After a night out, take off your clothes to reveal stockings and suspenders. (Even better, flash him a glimpse *while* you're out.)

- **Tease, tickle, and titillate.** Brush your lips over his mouth but don't let him kiss back. Put his penis momentarily in your mouth, then withdraw and start kissing his neck. Sit on top of him and let him partially penetrate you, then get up and walk away. The trick is to keep him unbelievably aroused rather than frustrated. At some point, though, you have to put him out of his misery by bringing things (and him) to a fabulous finale!

FIRST-TIME SEX AFTER A LONG-TERM LOVER

You've been out to every restaurant in town, they've been to your place, you've been to theirs, and now it's crunch time. Which is why you're in the bathroom, ostensibly cleaning your teeth (for the last twenty minutes) while your about-to-be-lover waits in the bedroom, wondering if you have any gums left. *Don't be ridiculous,* you lecture yourself in the mirror, *you've had sex hundreds, probably thousands of times before. Yeah,* says another little voice, *but with the same person for the last ten years.*

First-time sex with a new lover, after years with an old one, is heart-thumping stuff. Part of you can't wait to give it a whirl (no prizes for guessing *which* part), but the thinking bits would stay happily celibate for another one hundred years to avoid any embarrassment. But come out of that bathroom you must (the window's usually far too little to escape from). Just keep the following points in mind.

- **Don't panic if you feel as nervous as a virgin.** In a sense, it is like losing your virginity all over again. Don't fall into the same trap you did back then and expect that it's going to be wonderful. You've fantasized about it, so have they, and reality hasn't got a hope in hell of matching expectations.

- **Admit you are nervous.** If the thought of them gazing at your flesh makes you faint, leave your underwear on and slip under the sheets. Say, "I haven't had sex with anyone but Martha/Martin for years. I feel like a teenager." It'll ease the tension for both of you. You're not the only one who's under pressure. Your new lover feels they have to at least measure up to the standard set by your ex—and that's pretty difficult when your old lover's a few hundred practice runs ahead of them.

- **Stick to the basics.** If you're really nervous,

this is one situation where I advocate just getting through. Kiss, have some foreplay, do the deed. Get it over with, let most of your anxieties evaporate, *then* you can concentrate on getting to know each other properly (and don't be surprised if after all that fuss, you're actually keen for a repeat within the next half an hour).

- **If it's awful, admit it and laugh.** Say, "That was *such* a disaster because we were so nervous. But now that it's out of the way we can relax and really get to know each other sexually." It's not a big deal if she didn't lubricate or orgasm or if he couldn't get an erection, lost it, or came too quickly. It doesn't mean you're not compatible in bed. It doesn't mean you should have stuck it out with your ex. It just means you don't know each other's bodies, desires, or needs yet.

- **Accept that you may feel sad afterward.** For many people, especially women, sleeping with someone new marks the true ending of the previous relationship. It'll hit you like a lightning bolt: my God, it really is over. Even if you broke out the champagne when your ex left, don't be surprised if you have a postcoital grief attack. Cry, *sob* if you must, but don't shut your new lover out. If you're open and explain your emotions, they'll understand. Remember an ending is often the glorious beginning of something even better.

Dear Diary, I had sex today and it was . . .

Emma

Emma, 23, is single and living in Sydney. She works in the media and is bisexual, though doesn't classify herself as such. She says she's simply "nondiscriminatory" when it comes to

choosing a sex partner. Emma has had many lovers and several long-term relationships.

Week one

Ryan came over on Friday night and we went out to dinner then stayed up late talking. When we finally got to bed, it was already past 2 A.M. Ryan's a great friend and a wonderful lover—sensual, erotic, experienced, funny, relaxed. I love that controlled intensity of his. We fuck and it's good, but I don't come the first time and he knows this so he keeps touching me until I'm wet again. When he goes down on me, he knows exactly what he's doing and he enjoys doing it—an extra turn-on. He gets hard again and I put a condom on him using my mouth, which he finds very sexy. This time, when he makes love to me, I come and that makes him come, too. It's amazing. He sleeps over and when he finally leaves, I ask if he's got everything (he likes to leave his mark). Of course, he "forgets" a T-shirt that smells of his sweat and cologne and makes me horny, reminds me of him. I think about throwing it into the laundry with my stuff but end up sleeping with it under my pillow.

Later, I seduce myself, thinking about Ryan fucking me and going down on me with that great oral technique of his. Actually, I fantasize about other things, too, but I always like to imagine someone I know once I start to get aroused. It makes it more intimate. I wonder how he'd feel if he knew. He'd probably like to know I was thinking about him.

Week two

I'm in Melbourne on business and I meet Mark, a smart, sexy lawyer at a work function. There's an instant spark between us, one thing leads to another and I end up back at his apartment, in his bed. (Normally, I would have waited, but I'm flying back to Sydney tomorrow and I just can't resist!) Like most men, he's a little impatient and a tad heavy-handed at first, but I manage to convey my base-level requirements for enjoyable arousal and he does a pretty good job of fulfilling them. We fuck—using a condom that he provides—and it's sexy, athletic, and abandoned.

He goes down on me at one stage, quite expertly, and makes me extremely horny. Later, we do it "doggie" and by the time he comes (loudly, which is great—I like his lack of inhibition and sense of theatrics), I'm so turned on that I only have to touch myself for thirty seconds or so and I also orgasm (not quite as loudly, which is probably just as well). We doze, cozily entwined, his hard body against my soft flesh. At seven, far too early, it's time to go. I leave him sleeping, again a stranger, creep into last night's clothes and steal away, leaving nothing but a hastily penned phone number and a kiss.

Today I miss Stephen, my ex, once the love of my life. Back in Sydney, I go to see a film by myself and it makes me nostalgic and miss him more. I want a love with intensity. I want to feel that strongly again, to fuck someone I would die for, someone I'd want to get pregnant with. Someone I'd miss. My friend Max calls and he's sweet and concerned but I don't feel passion for him. He's a darling, though, and it will be good to see him. I could use some steadying. I could use some more sex, too.

Week three

I'm at work and a big bouquet of tiny pink roses arrives from Mark. I call to thank him and we arrange to catch up next time I'm in town. He's great on the phone—he's got a really sexy English accent—but I shouldn't think this way when I'm in the office. I can't wait to go to Melbourne again.

I have spent the last twenty-four hours on a hot date at home. Max came over and we cooked Italian, drank a bottle of good red, and watched a steamy video. It was quite good but I lost attention halfway through when Max took his shirt off. It was a shameless bid for my attention—and it worked. Great body. He used to have a hairy back and a white, pasty torso that reminded me of uncooked bread. But he waxes now, works out, and goes to the tanning salon. He's too young but utterly charming and seductive, witty, quick, manually dexterous, and great around the house. Kind of a nice package, don't you think? I was quite happy to go along with everything he suggested (again). I didn't like anal sex much before Max but he uses his fingers and tongue-fucks my anus and for the first time, I actually contemplated having his penis inside my rectum. It's very addictive, what he does. Ryan called on my machine as Max was licking me and that was such a turn-on: hearing one guy on my machine saying how much he wanted me while another gives me the licking of my life. Max doesn't want me as his; we're just friends who fuck. He didn't put his shirt back on until 8:30 the *following* evening. Yum.

Ryan calls, just for a chat. We arrange to go out together next week and easily slip into friendship mode. He's the perfect escort—polite, sociable, good looking, and he wears fantastic designer clothes. There's no guarantee we'll end up in bed together after our date and even if we do, we'll probably just cuddle and go to sleep. We're more friends than lovers really. Both of us know we're not soul mates but we're extremely fond of each other and I can imagine us being friends for life. If only more men were like him—most want to own you or run away.

Week four

I feel really horny tonight—it's that time of the month. I get out the trusty vibrator, read some porn to get off, go for quantity rather than quality. It's fun even though it's tacky. At least it stops me from climbing the walls, gets the circulation going, and I wake up satisfied. Guys—who needs them?

I've always slept with women and can't really imagine why anyone would write off half the population sexually just because they're the same sex. So when Natasha and I stay in, cooking dinner, dancing to the stereo, trying on clothes, it's natural that I start to feel horny. She comes up and starts stroking me and it feels sensual, comfortable, and at the same time, very exciting. Girls having sex is still such a taboo it always gives me an illicit thrill. We kiss and her mouth is so soft, it couldn't possibly be a man. Both of us are horny but we take it slowly, like two sleepy cats. Going down on her is warm and erotic. As always, it makes me understand how guys feel—it isn't easy to give good head to a girl! I stop before she comes and she kisses me everywhere.

We end up with our legs entwined and come that way. It's wild and wonderful and the best thing is, when it's over, we go back to being two girlfriends having a cozy evening. No pressure. No intimacy. I like girls, they have their own special charm, but I don't fall in love with them.

It's morning and I'm in Melbourne for the week. I'm at Mark's, trying to write this, and he's being very provocative. Later, maybe—or maybe really soon. He's shaping up rather nicely—lived up to the few phone calls we've had and we haven't stopped having sex since I got here. It's weird, the more sex I have, the more I need it and the less it seems to matter who it's with.

My sex life is . . . Exciting and satisfying—although I have my disappointments like everyone else. I know this diary makes me sound like I always have fantastic sex but I think you just caught me at a wild, wonderful time of my life. I guess you would say I'm promiscuous if you counted the number of lovers I've had, but I don't think I sleep around at all. I pick my lovers very carefully because sex is extremely, extremely important to me. It's one of the most important things in my life and I put a great deal of energy into it. I'm definitely in tune with my body and my needs. Some of my friends say they envy my sex life but I think anyone can have great sex if they just learn to let go, relax, and really listen to what their body is telling them. They seem so hung up on what their lovers will think if they do this or that. I say, forget the lovers, satisfy yourself first!

Steamy Stuff

••

If you're not good at giving oral sex (even worse, can't be bothered learning), give up now on ever graduating from sex school. Nothing will score you more points than delivering mind-blowing fellatio (the posh term for giving him oral sex) or cunnilingus (ditto for her). Oral sex is the one erotic act everyone consistently reports wanting more of. If being told "You're a great lay" is a compliment, you'll be worshipped for performing hellishly good head-jobs!

THE 10-STEP GUIDE TO THE BEST FELLATIO HE'S EVER HAD

Giving him mind-blowing fellatio is number one on his sex wish list, and it's the thing most women feel least confident about. Who better to ask for tips than a sex worker who specializes in it? (If you have something against taking advice from experienced, high-class sex workers, get over it now. They make a living out of sex and are experts in their field.) I asked Olivia, a skilled fellatrix, to reveal her most intimate secrets for this no-holds-barred guide to giving him pleasure. Prepare to turn from the most nervous novice into an instant expert—and have him begging for more! This is her guide, so I'll let her tell you in her own words . . .

1. Learn to love it

"Women who love sex are good at it; it's as simple as that. If you don't like giving him oral sex, the best techniques in the world won't turn you into a skilled fellatrix. Usually it's the smell, swallowing, or gagging that women are scared of and all are easily fixed. Turn a shower into foreplay if he's not scrupulously clean and use the soap as a lubricant to masturbate his penis (if he's uncircumcised pull the foreskin back very gently and wash underneath). Gagging isn't a problem if you use my techniques, and you don't have to swallow to be good at oral sex.

"Fellatio, or 'French' as we call it, is requested and enjoyed by almost all clients, regardless of the sex worker's speciality. Show him that you love doing it—make lots of noise and '*uuumms*,' compliment him on his penis—and he'll be any-thing *but* putty in your hands! Get to know his penis: examine it, talk about it. Be aware of his body language. Learn how to read his moods and play up to any secret fantasies."

2. Give him lots of foreplay

"Women aren't the only ones who love foreplay (even if *he* hasn't realized it yet) and your mouth shouldn't be anywhere near his penis till it's rock hard. Pamper him by giving him a massage, then a 'body tease.' Oil his body and yours and lie over him, supporting your weight on your hands. Come in close and slide up and down, gyrate your pelvis against his body letting him feel how turned on you are, and push your bottom in the air (especially if there's a mirror behind you). If you've got long hair, use it; lean forward and let it caress his body. Bite his nipples, and tease him by lowering yourself over his penis so your genitals are touching but don't let him penetrate. Give him 'Spanish': put his penis between your breasts and roll and knead them around it using your hands. Stroke, lick, and nibble your way down his body while you're telling him exactly what you're about to do to him. Get feedback: ask him what *he'd* like you to do."

3. Vary the scene and stimulate all his senses

"Don't do it in the same position every time. Guys love getting oral sex just about anywhere, but variety's a turn-on. Try him standing up and you kneeling or squatting in front of him; him up against a wall; a '69er'; in the car; in the park while walking home from a restaurant.

> "Most girls, they treat your penis like a lollipop. Licking alone doesn't do a thing for me and most of the time they'll screw up their faces during oral sex, like it's some nasty object. You know she's only doing it because she thinks you expect her to. That's why if you meet a girl who gets off on giving head, you're stoked."
> Danny, 18, gym instructor

Different locations add a fresh psychological kick. It doesn't matter what you're wearing, but lots of men find it exciting if you're totally naked and he's fully clothed with just his zip undone; alternatively, try you fully dressed and him totally naked. Make sure he can watch. Men are erotic visualists and primarily aroused by what they can see, one reason why they're so into girlie mags. He'll want to see your face, maybe even hold your hair back. Don't close your eyes, keep them open. I hold eye contact with the man while I'm fellating him and make 'horny eyes'—narrow them sexily and make them smolder. If you're too embarrassed to look at him, look at his penis instead."

4. Don't just concentrate on his penis

"His anus, perineum, testicles—all are erogenous zones you should pay attention to before and during fellatio. Get him to lie on his back then lick and stroke him on the perineum (the area between his anus and testicles), massaging it with slight pressure. Bend his legs back and lick from the base of his anus through to the scrotum. Cradle his testicles in your hand, lick them, take one or both in your mouth. Massage near the base of his penis, one hand holding it, the other massaging."

5. Use your hands and start masturbating him

"Always use two hands during oral sex: one to stimulate him elsewhere (nipples, testicles, anus), the other as a guide. It gives you more control and he can't gag you. I usually keep one hand at the bottom of the shaft of his penis, then it's up to me to control how deeply I take it into my mouth. Lots of men like to put their hands on the back of your head, but tell him it's hands-*off* if he won't stop pushing you deeper than you want to go. 'Deep-throating' is a head game more than anything else. If you can do it, great! If you can't or don't want to, rest assured that it doesn't necessarily feel better; it's just what he's seen in a porn film. Most feeling is at the head of his penis not the bottom. If you're really paranoid about gagging, place the penis to one side of your mouth rather than dead center."

6. Take control of his penis but handle with care

"Some women are too rough! The best way to find out how he likes being masturbated is to get him to show you how he does it himself, then imitate the technique. Don't tug or yank at his foreskin if he's uncircumcised; make sure it slides up and over the penile head. Take a firm grip, then start teasing. Let him see your nice pink tongue and play up the lick movements. Do long, lollipop licks, lick up the side, around the head, cover your

Is it fattening? There are around 36 calories in the average ejaculate of sperm, while about 150 calories are burned in an hour of sex.

teeth with your lips (and keep them that way!), and do 'lip-pinches' (a biting motion without teeth involved) up and down the side of the shaft. Use lots of saliva: the more lubricated he is, the more pleasurable it will feel. Finally, take his penis right into your mouth, swirl your tongue around the head, then withdraw and give a big 'uuummm' of satisfaction!"

7. Technique is all-important

"The basic technique is to slide your hand up and down his penis (closing it when you reach the head, opening it slightly as you slide down the length) as it's moving in and out of your mouth. With your lips covering your teeth, close your mouth around the penis and encircle it so there's a firm but comfortable pressure. You're not actually sucking, you're more making sure your mouth is a snug fit. Practice on your finger and imagine it's his penis. What sort of sensations seem like they'd feel good? Imagine how his penis feels when it's in your vagina and try to imitate the sensation. When you're confident, move into the 'twist-and-swirl': make a gentle twisting motion with your hand as you're sliding it up and down his penis and swirl your tongue around the rim of the head, paying particular attention to the frenulum (the small piece of skin where the head meets the shaft). Tense your tongue and vibrate it; swirl it around the head and the base—the more tongue movements while it's in your mouth the better! As with women, a steady rhythm is important. Start off agonizingly slow, then increase the pressure and the rhythm as he approaches orgasm."

8. Tease him mercilessly

"Take him to the brink of orgasm (you'll get better at timing this with practice!) so he experiences that intensely pleasurable preorgasm wave several times, then stop fellating him and use your mouth on his testes, the perineum, and his anus before returning. Be creative and use different strokes: long slides up and down his penis, taking it deep in your mouth; shorter strokes concentrating on the head and inserting just the tip. Once he's approaching orgasm, however, stick with the same technique and rhythm."

9. Step up the stimulation just as he's about to orgasm

"The male G-spot is about one to two inches inside the anus and by inserting a finger, you'll make his orgasm even more intense. If he enjoys anal stimulation, he'll push his bottom toward you or stick it up in the air the minute you start to explore the area. Be gentle and make sure your finger is well lubricated. If you feel uncomfortable doing this, give him a stronger orgasm by pressing the perineum area firmly with your thumb as he's ejaculating."

If his sperm tastes bad, it could be something he ate. What he eats and drinks hours before making love strongly affects the way he tastes. For the best flavored sperm, feed him bland foods like pasta and potatoes; for the worst, serve a curry, washed down with beer and coffee.

10. Decide beforehand what you'll do when he ejaculates

"It will be obvious when he's about to orgasm: the penis starts to throb, jerk, and spasm; some men stop thrusting and stay perfectly still, others thrust harder. Some men are oversensitive when they orgasm so keep your hands away from the head of the penis and masturbate him at the bottom. If you're going to swallow his semen, do it properly. Don't make faces; simply swallow it and say 'yuuumm.' If you don't want to, don't take any sperm in your mouth; spitting it out is rude, unattractive, and insulting. Instead, withdraw when he's in the throes of orgasm and continue stimulating him with your hand. A sexy alternative to swallowing is to let him ejaculate elsewhere on your body—over your breasts or your neck. If you rub it into your body afterward, he'll know you enjoyed fellating him as much as he enjoyed receiving it!"

TRICKS OF THE TRADE

- **Drink a hot drink beforehand.** The sensation of a hot mouth around his penis is sensational! Smearing honey or cream over it, then licking it off, adds a fun element.
- **Play up to the power fantasy.** Power—having it or being completely dominated—is a common fantasy for many men. Let him

call the shots and kneel before him or *you* take control and let him know you're boss!

- **Clean your tongue with a toothbrush** every time you clean your teeth. A healthy, pink tongue is a turn-on.

- **If he goes limp, slow it down.** Ask him why. Either he's stressed or tired and can't concentrate or you're not fellating him correctly. Applying too much pressure—holding him too tightly with your hand or sucking too hard—can make him lose his erection. Also bear in mind that men are individuals with their own preferred turn-ons and techniques. Talk, start again, and slow it down.

- **To make him orgasm quickly** insert a finger into his anus or press the perineum firmly with your thumb. The more extra stimulation you give, the quicker he'll usually orgasm.

- **It's what you do before** your mouth even touches his penis that counts. The more foreplay and teasing he's had, the more sensitive he'll be. Just about any sensation will feel great!

THE 10-STEP GUIDE TO OHMIGOD-DON'T-EVER-STOP ORAL SEX FOR HER

Cunnilingus is the rather unexotic name for you giving her oral sex, but men who master it rarely lack lovers. Trouble is, it's *dark* down there and you're often forced to rely on touch and feel rather than eyesight. Apart from eating more carrots, there's not too much you can do about the natural lighting around her vagina. But you can persuade her to let you turn the lights on because it's essential you get this technique right. With some women, oral sex is the only way you'll get her to reach orgasm; for the rest, it's often the most intense. Again, I went to an expert to find out how best to perform cunnilingus. David is a male escort and sex worker who only services women. And guess what's the most com-

> Oral sex has officially replaced intercourse as a female's favorite sexual activity—well, it certainly has in one American college. Ninety-six percent of the thousand female students surveyed claimed they enjoyed cunnilingus more than penetration.

monly requested thing on his menu? Here, in his words, are his professional tips. Don't just read this section, *study* it. If you want to make her quiver, this is how!

1. Women are slower to become aroused and slower to reach orgasm than men, so time—not rushing her—is the biggest luxury you can give a woman

"If she's stressed, relax her first by massaging or stroking her body until she starts to become aroused. Follow this with lots of kissing on the neck, and stroke and lick her breasts and nipples before moving on to her genitals. Leave her underwear on and stroke her through the fabric until she becomes wet; only then remove it."

2. Start by running your hands up and down the outside, then the inside of her thighs and at this point, ask her how she likes oral sex: slow, fast, gentle, or hard

"While kissing and licking down her body, pull the outer vaginal lips over the inner ones in a gentle, circular motion to warm the entire area."

3. Position counts

"If she's shy, it's best if she lies back while you're kneeling at the foot of the bed between her legs. Lots of women love being licked while they're standing and you're kneeling (it appeals to their slave fantasies, plus they can control the pressure and rhythm by holding your head) or being licked from behind. Another favorite that gives her ultimate control: lie back on the bed while she kneels above you and lowers her genitals down to your mouth. She may put her hands flat against the wall behind for balance. Some women like to feel completely exposed with their legs wide open, others prefer their legs quite closely wrapped around your head. It all depends on how sensitive her clitoris is."

> "I stayed with a complete loser of a guy for six months simply because he gave the best oral sex I'd had in my life. I was addicted to it. I couldn't give him up because—and sadly, this is true so far— I knew I'd never find a tongue like that again."
> Mary, 24, secretary

4. It's really important to keep her moist, so use lots of saliva to lick the entire area before concentrating on the clitoris

"Don't tense or point your tongue; it is better to use the whole surface of the flat of your tongue rather than just the tip. That's the one thing that most men do wrong. Start with indirect stimulation, gently wiggling your tongue around and over the clitoris: it's toward the top of the vagina and feels like a tiny marble."

5. Move into longer, wet, gentle strokes with your tongue, keeping up a slow but steady rhythm

"Rhythm is really important; chopping and changing techniques and rhythm all the time doesn't work with women. Read her body language or ask her what stroke feels best, then keep on doing it. If she pulls away, you're being too rough; if she presses her vagina closer or pulls your head closer, step up the pressure slightly."

6. It's generally best to be too gentle than too rough

"Again, ask her what feels best. Try shaking your head from side to side, making circles around the edge of the clitoris as well as up-and-down strokes."

7. Make sure she knows how much you are enjoying yourself by making noise

"If she thinks you're enjoying it as much as she is, she relaxes and knows she can take her time. Again, you have to be prepared to settle in and keep going until she says to stop. The tongue movements are gentle and if a guy can't keep them up for at least ten to fifteen minutes, his tongue's too tense or he's doing it too fast."

8. When she's really aroused, insert a finger inside her vagina

"A lot of women like to be inserted with a finger or dildo just before orgasm but others find it distracting. If she's good at communicating, she'll pull your hand away if she doesn't like it; if she does, she'll usually move her hips against your hand to achieve deeper penetration. Some women like manually stimulating their own clitorises while you're performing oral sex; others put their fingers down to feel your tongue working on them. If she does either, lick her fingers as well."

9. *When you're not manually masturbating her as well as licking, use your other hand to knead her breasts and nipples or to stroke the perineum, the area between her anus and vagina*

"Some women like a lubricated finger inserted into their anus as they orgasm; try inserting the tip gently and see if she pulls away before going any deeper."

"It's weird, but I don't really like guys giving me head. I don't know why, I just feel uncomfortable. I'm not prudish about anything else. I've only ever liked it with one guy—and he was so good, he had a reputation for giving great oral sex. Somehow he hit all the right spots. With everyone else, though, I can take it or leave it. Leave it really."
Nikki, 17, student

10. Her body will tense when she's close to orgasm

"At this point, increase the pressure slightly or move a little faster. The most important thing, though, is to maintain the rhythm as best you can even if she starts moving around. As she's actually orgasming, switch back to slow, gentle strokes but make sure you cover the whole clitoral area by using the whole surface of your tongue. Most women's clitorises are unbearably sensitive immediately after an orgasm, so don't be surprised if she puts a hand down to cover it or pushes your head away."

THE FIVE THINGS MOST MEN DO WRONG

1. **You only do it if we ask and obviously find it off-putting.** A man who turns his nose up and says "it smells," even when she's fresh out of the shower, is being ridiculous. Assuming she doesn't have any infections, the natural scent of a vagina is musky and sensual. Don't blame her for swapping lovers if you can't be convinced.

2. **You're too rough.** Some women like a very firm tongue, but gentle suits most of us. The clitoris is sensitive, so while overenthusiastic licking will have her squirming, it's with pain, not pleasure.

3. **You don't do it for long enough.** You might be able to orgasm at the mere sight of her mouth wrapped around your penis, but she takes longer to climax. Tell her she can take as long as she wants because you *love* doing it to her and she's yours for life.

4. **You change techniques too often.** Women need regular, consistent rhythm for an extended period in order to orgasm. While she might be impressed with your extensive repertoire of mouth movements, stick with one or two each session. The clitoris is a funny beast—it can be terribly turned on by one sensation, but take ages to get used to another if you chop and change.

5. **You stop at the crucial moment.** You might like stimulation to stop while you're orgasming, but we prefer it to continue, though often softer, right through to the

last spasm. If you stop just as we're hovering on the brink, we often don't make it over the fence.

Dear Diary, I had sex today and it was . . .

Jane
Jane, 32, has been seeing Brad, 27, for the past ten months. Jane finds it difficult to trust men and has not had a relationship that's lasted more than three months since she was 18. Brad's clocked up four long-term lovers. They describe their relationship as "shaky at best."

Week one
I resigned from my job yesterday, which was pretty nerve-racking because I'd been working there for five years. During the day, while I was waiting to see my boss, I made half a dozen phone calls to Brad so he could reassure me about what I was doing. He's very good at boosting my self-confidence. When I finally rang to tell him I'd done it, he told me he'd booked us into a five-star hotel for the night. We spent the

night drinking champagne, eating room service food, and making love. Brad's also very good at that. He's the only one who's ever been able to make me orgasm.

I don't know why, but I've always been uptight about sex. In my wild days, I used to hang around with a few girlfriends who I guess were quite promiscuous and I started to take a more recreational view of sex. It was probably quite good for me, but I started having one-night stands like they did and they hurt too much and put me off sex again. My friends were seriously in it for the sex, but I only wanted the affection. I fell in love all the time.

Week two

My stress level's cranked up to maximum. I'm worried about whether I've done the right thing switching jobs, I've got work projects due, and I'm paranoid about the weight I've put on since I gave up smoking. All of which means I don't feel particularly desirable or desiring of sex. Brad always says he doesn't want me to feel as though I have to make love, but sometimes, like Thursday, I do even when I don't feel like it. It felt awful. I was so dry he can't have enjoyed it but I don't think he should pay just because I'm having a bad week.

Week three

This week was the worst on record. I start a new job then get the flu. Unfortunately, it's a bad week for Brad, too. I want attention, he wants attention. So we both get it by arguing with each other—constantly. The end result is that we haven't made love in eight days. Even though I'm not that fussed about sex, it makes me feel close to him. It's like the chicken and the egg thing: I can't feel close to him until we have sex, but we can't because I don't feel close. Figure that out.

Week four

All we've done is take turns at ending the relationship. One day we argue and I call it off. Then he backpedals and it's on again. The next day, it's his turn to end it and I do the apologizing. Last night, I told him I wanted him to sleep in the spare room. That's because I can deceive myself very easily when I'm asleep or half-asleep and pretend everything is okay. Ever since we started sharing a bed, we've been a very cuddly couple. In the middle of the night, I'll sometimes wake up and Brad is putting his arms around me and telling me he loves me. Even when we're fighting, I'll wake up to discover I'm wrapped around him and I forget about being angry. We did end up sleeping together in the end, but that's all we did. I don't think we touched each other all night and then, this morning, he just got up and left. I'm scared. Where do we go now?

My sex life is . . . Sadly over for the moment! We're definitely off and I have no hope it will be on again. It's a shame because this was the best sex I'd ever had in terms of physical sensations. The touchy-feely side of the relationship was pretty good, too. But we really are different personalities: he's laid-back and easygoing, I'm someone whose button is permanently stuck on fast-forward. I always wanted to move forward, he wanted to stop and smell the roses. Perhaps that's why he was so good in bed and I'm not.

3

Hot and Sweaty

....

There are more than six hundred docu-
mented positions for intercourse and
you'd be asleep within minutes if I tried to
list each one of them. Instead, I'm going to
focus on the five favorite positions before
going bottom-up, then trumpeting the case
for the much-maligned quickie and finally
suggesting a totally new way to have penetra-
tive sex. Sounds intriguing? It is. But whatever position or technique you do, promise
me you'll do it with passion. Both of you will
get a lot more out of all that humping and

grinding if you thrust your hips to meet each other's, grab bottoms and pull them close to you, run your hands up and down backs, arms, and backs of thighs, or lick or bite the closest thing to your mouths. Go for it. Make so much noise, your neighbors consider double-glazing their windows!

THE FIVE FAVORITE POSITIONS

Despite the endless variety possible, the average couple alternates between two or three positions, most settling on missionary, woman-on-top, and rear-entry. There's no such thing as "the best" position—it all depends on your shape and height, your individual preferences and mood at the time. Some positions work well if he comes too soon; side-by-side suits lazy, Sunday-morning sex; and rear-entry is good for a fast and furious "quickie."

For most men, orgasm is guaranteed in just about any (if not all) intercourse positions. For women (sigh!), as I said, it's a different story. Clitoral stimulation is pretty well an essential for most of us to come during intercourse, so

I've not only addressed this section to women but included "Orgasm potential for her" under each position. But don't be too concerned if your partner's favorite position is different from yours or vice versa; take it in turns or do both in the same session.

Missionary

Rumor has it that early missionaries, sent to "civilize" the colonies, considered this the only respectable way to make love. Hence the name "missionary" position and its rather staid image.

It was probably the first position in which you had intercourse. I suspect it'll be the last (bodies aren't too agile at ninety) and, even if we hate to admit it, it's how most couples have intercourse most of the time. For good reason. The basic position—the woman lying on her back, legs apart with the man between them—requires zero imagination, little effort on her part, and is reasonably comfortable for both. It's the position you use when you're both fairly interested in sex but not spinning cartwheels over it. Ironically, it's also the first position to spring to mind when you're so eager for him to be inside you, you don't care how the hell he does it, as long as he does it *now*. Missionary also appeals to the come-on-you've-got-to-admit-I've-put-on-weight girl (that is, 99 percent of women) because of the flat-tummy thing. We lie on our backs, the flab spreads out, and we look extra thin. Bonus!

> "I don't come during intercourse but I love it all the same. It makes me feel close to my boyfriend. Our bodies fit together, it's all wet and hard, and I feel all filled up. The initial thrust is always the best, especially if we've teased each other to the point where neither of us can wait any longer."
> Naomi, 25, secretary

Why it feels good for her

You're face-to-face and can talk and kiss, so it can be quite romantic. But you also have less control over what's happening and basically can't move very far. Bend your knees for deeper

> "I'd say most guys would nominate missionary or rear-entry as their favorite positions. The first one's easy and no effort; in the second, you're guaranteed to get your rocks off. Doggie was also the position I most enjoyed when I was with a girl I loved. I think I now associate it with her and the good times."
> Steve, 24, gym instructor

penetration. Stimulate the clitoris more effectively by keeping your legs together (squeezing your thighs) and have his legs open, lying over the *outside* of yours.

Why it feels good for him

He basically runs the show, being in complete control of the depth of penetration, the angle, and the pace. For this reason, it's not a bad choice if he's a premature ejaculator because he can stop if he gets too carried away. If the opposite's the problem (he's had one drink too many and having trouble orgasming), reach down and hold back the skin on his penis, grasping at the root of the shaft with your finger and thumb, while he's moving in and out of you. There is one drawback for both of you: neither of you can see any of the real action.

Orgasm potential for her
It's not great for manual stimulation of your clitoris, but it can make him last longer in intercourse if that's a problem.

How to make it even better
Put one or two hard pillows under your bottom; pull your knees up to your chest or wrap them around his back for deeper penetration; try lifting your legs high and resting one or both feet on his shoulders; lie sideways and move most of your body off the bed, head resting on a cushion on the floor (yes, the blood will rush to your head but that's the idea—some women swear this makes female orgasms scream material).

One way to make it instantly more exciting for both of you is to put a ban on using the missionary position. If you do "slip up" (and you will—anything "banned" becomes immediately desirable), it'll seem naughty, forbidden, and anything but boring.

How to vary it

Get him to stimulate your G-spot. Rather than thrusting in and out, you half sit up, lift your bottom, then slowly lean backward, repeat until one (or both) of you climax; let him lift your legs up and hold them; roll over completely and end up with—you on top!

Comfort rating for him

His arms can get tired supporting his own weight.

Comfort rating for her

Unless he rests his weight on his elbows or hands and knees, even breathing can be difficult. If he's the size of a sumo wrestler and you're a waif, forget it.

Woman-on-top

Any woman worth her stuff, in or out of bed, has to revel in this one, even if it's just for the connotations of the name. You on top, you in control—it's deliciously *liberated*, not to mention a hell of a turn-on for both of you. For best control and balance, most women sit on top of their partner, who's lying on his back, then lower themselves onto his penis, legs bent at the knees and folded backward. You can also try squatting. In the basic position, you're usually facing him. Don't try woman-on-top unless he's very hard—it's incredibly easy to bend a semierect penis and cause injury.

Number of positions in which most couples have intercourse: two to five. The favorites: missionary and woman-on-top. Percentage of lovers who use more than twenty positions regularly: 5 percent.

Why it feels good for her

It's the opposite to the missionary: instead of him calling the shots, you have complete control over the depth of penetration, angle, and speed. You're in the power position and can show off all you like. Exhibitionists don't do it any other way, but even if you're not one, it's still fantastic. (If you don't feel confident about showing off your body, simply lean forward.) If deep penetration sometimes hurts—your cervix is sensitive for instance—this is one position you can relax in, without fear of pain. He can only go as deep as you let him.

Why it feels good for him

He gets off on watching your body and what's happening—this position lays it all right in front of him. He can see your body clearly and watch the expressions on your face as you approach orgasm. *You* might think breasts look ridiculous wobbling up and down, *he* thinks they look sexy. Not only that, he gets the double bonus of watching his penis disappear into your vagina while you do all the work. The pressure's off. You're looking after your own pleasure (at least in terms of penetration), and he doesn't have to worry about timing or depth.

Orgasm potential for her

Both his hands are free to caress your breasts and stimulate the clitoris (lean forward and lift up a little for easier access). If you're a fan of the G-spot, this position is likely to hit it (lean backward). It's also pretty easy for you to touch your own clitoris and bring yourself to orgasm while he's inside you.

How to make it even better

Try moving in small circles as you're lifting yourself up and down; tease him a little (or a lot) by rubbing his erect penis over your vaginal lips, letting him enter just a fraction then denying him full penetration by lifting tantalizingly higher; turn him on by playing with your own breasts or your clitoris.

How to vary it

Face his toes instead of his head (resist the urge to do a 180-

> "I *hate* getting on top. My legs seize up, I feel stupid, and it hurts my back. I also hate doggie. It makes me feel cheap and undignified."
> Louise, 32, real estate saleswoman

degree turn while impaled unless you warn him first); get him to hold your waist to help you move up and down; lean forward or backward to experience the sensation of stimulation on different parts of your vaginal walls; lie (instead of sitting or crouching) on top of him with your legs outside or inside his; try him sitting in a chair with you on his lap; try him sitting up with legs straight out in front of him, you lower yourself onto his penis and sit with your knees bent and feet flat on the floor.

Comfort rating for him
Ten out of ten—what's *not* to like? Women are usually lighter than men, so he's unlikely to complain about you being too heavy.

Comfort rating for her
It can be tiring if you're using your legs to move up and down, but think of it this way: you can skip the squat machine at the gym the next day.

Rear-entry (or "doggie-style")

This position allows *deep* penetration and ignites the animal instinct in anyone with a libido because it's so primitive. It's a firm favorite with any couple who really get into sex, and is avoided by couples who think walking hand-in-hand along a beach is racy. A warning for women with men who come too soon: don't even let him think about this one unless you're both happy with a quickie. With the combination of deep penetration, the unleashing of the "beast" in him because he's "taking you," fantasies soaring right off the pleasure scale because he can't see your face and could be having sex with anyone . . . He'll last, *ooohh*, two seconds if you're lucky.

Men used to initiate sex 75 percent of the time, now women are the first to suggest it 40 percent of the time.

Why it feels good for her

Uninhibited women love rear-entry—anyone with a slave fantasy can let their imagination run riot (rear-entry is him at his most dominant and you at your most submissive and vulnerable). Because you can't see him, he could be anyone (the guy on your favorite soap, the wonderfully *built* workman you saw on the street, your boyfriend's best friend). Your breasts are often hanging down so the blood flows to the nipples and makes them extra sensitive.

Why it feels good for him

It allows him to penetrate as deeply as he possibly can and he's visually stimulated (turned on by what he can see more than by what he can feel). The sight of his penis pumping in and out of your vagina is, well . . . his idea of heaven really. Your bottom presses against his testicles for extra stimulation and speaking of bottoms, most men *love* being able to see yours. (No, he's not looking at how "fat" it is.)

Orgasm potential for her

Orgasms often feel more intense because he's hitting the sensitive bits (the front wall of your vagina). His hands are totally free to stimulate your breasts from behind or your clitoris.

This is by far the best position to stimulate the G-spot since the penis hits the front vaginal wall directly.

How to make it even better
Give in totally and let him penetrate you from behind while you're on all fours.

How to vary it
Rather than kneel: you lie facedown, flat on the bed, legs spread, he lies on top of you and penetrates from behind (great for indirectly stimulating the clitoris). Try him standing behind you, you stand then lean forward until your hands touch the floor. Attempt "the wheelbarrow": he stands behind you, then lifts and holds your straight legs like a wheelbarrow while you've got your weight supported on your elbows on the bed.

Comfort rating for him
He's a prime target for carpet burn on the knees if you're doing it on the living room floor but does he care? Nah!

Comfort rating for her

Rear-entry positions allow deep penetration—too deep sometimes, especially if he gets completely carried away and starts thrusting like he's trying to find oil. If it feels too deep, lift your bottom. Better still, simply ask him to hold back and go shallower.

Face-to-face positions while sitting or kneeling

Close and intimate, many people find these positions a relaxing variation on the norm. Positions where you're sitting on the end of the bed, he's kneeling in front of you on the floor; you sitting in his lap while he also sits up—these are all examples of what the sexperts call "face-to-face." They're good for adding variety and are relatively easy to move into from missionary or woman-on-top since most are derivatives of these anyway.

Why it feels good for her

They're versatile, there's good eye contact, and he's in the ideal position to hold his penis and use it to manually masturbate your clitoris and vaginal lips.

Why it feels good for him

You can put your hands behind him and pull him to you by grabbing his buttocks. He'll like the visual stimulation of watching your genitals do their stuff.

The shower, the kitchen table, the living-room floor, and behind a locked bathroom door at crowded parties—these are the places five hundred women said they'd prefer to make love in. Anywhere but the bedroom.

Orgasm potential for her

In most positions, he can see and touch the clitoris easily, making it easy for him to masturbate you to orgasm.

How to make it even better

Try rocking as you're thrusting, using your legs as leverage to maintain a steady rhythm.

How to vary it

Use it to spice up your "favorites." Change into a face-to-face sitting position from woman-on-top or missionary, even if it's just for a few moments.

Comfort rating for him
Your heights and sizes can make some positions difficult, even impossible. Don't choose a position that he feels "twisted" in if he's got back problems or if you're a bigger person than he is.

Comfort rating for her
Some women complain of leg cramps but if you share the work—sometimes he thrusts, sometimes you do—it shouldn't be a problem.

Side-by-side
It's comfortable, cuddly, and sensual—perfect for those languid days when you're nicely turned on but not frothing at the mouth to get it. The favorite is the "spoon" (nicknamed because the shape the two of you make is rather like a pair of spoons nestled together). You lie on your side, he enters you from behind, arms wrapped around you. Draw your knees up to allow him to penetrate, then keep your bottom

stuck out toward him and the top knee forward.

Why it feels good for her

There's lots of body contact, and both his hands are free to play with your breasts, neck, and clitoris. It's very cuddly and effortless if you're tired or not very well.

Why it feels good for him

It's great for premature ejaculators because it's less "full-on" but also comfortable enough for him to settle in and take his time orgasming. There's maximum body contact and it's easy for her to reach behind and caress your buttocks, testicles, or perineum.

Orgasm potential for her

Hit the G-spot by getting him to lean back and away from you diagonally. It's easy for him to reach around and use his fingers to stimulate your clitoris.

How to make it even better

Turn it into an X: your heads are at opposite ends of the bed and you're making an X with your legs, he's inside you, each of you has one leg underneath each other's, one above. Clasp hands for control; this is great for slowing him down if he ejaculates too quickly.

How to vary it

Grind your bottom against his penis, bending from the waist and moving your upper torso downward. Reach around to fondle his penis while it's moving in and out of you.

Comfort rating for him

For relaxed, unhurried lovemaking it's a winner all-round.

Comfort rating for her

Ditto. It's also more comfortable than him-on-top positions if your partner is heavy. A bonus for both of you—you can fall asleep in exactly the same position you made love in.

BOTTOMS UP! A GUIDE TO ANAL STIMULATION

Our bottoms are "forbidden" zones, so the naughty element (if-I-can't-do-it-I-must) makes anal stimulation automatically exciting for many people. Quite apart from the psychological kick, the anus and rectum in both sexes are packed with nerve endings. For some, it's their most highly charged erogenous zone.

But for every couple that adores adding anal stimulation to their lovemaking, particularly during intercourse, there's another that turns pale at the mere idea of someone touching them in their most "private" spot. For that reason, I wouldn't advise anyone to pounce on their partner, airily promising the best sensation they've ever had, without telling them exactly where they plan to stick their finger first. If your partner blanches at the prospect, that's their choice, and it's not up to you to change their mind. However you *can* gently point out that if they're worried about it being messy, they needn't be. The lower rectum is normally empty and as long as fingers are clean and well lubricated with nails trimmed, they're not going to cause any damage. (Inserting *objects* into the rectum is another story. We don't want you the laughingstock of the hospital emergency room, do we?) Washing your hands thoroughly afterward, *before* touching her vagina or his penis, protects against any transference of bacteria.

"The first time a lover put his finger up my bottom, I was absolutely horrified. He gave no prewarning, just shoved it up there with no lubrication. I hated it but it's a different story with the guy I'm seeing now. He knows when and how to do it properly and now I can't orgasm unless he penetrates me anally."
Sue, 26, mother

The feelings produced by anal stimulation are quite different than what you're used to and it's great for heightening sensations you're already experiencing. Combine it with intercourse and your orgasms will feel exquisitely erotic; you can also use it during oral sex or while mutually masturbating each other. Simultaneous clitoral and anal stimulation makes both feel even better; insert a finger during intercourse to give him an exceptional climax.

If this is your first time, I'd try the following exercise during oral sex or mutual masturbation first, then introduce it during intercourse. It's a bit hard to keep thrusting away *and* ask questions and gently explore the area at the same time. Get to know each other's "yes" and "no-thanks-very-much" spots first, then try it just as your partner approaches orgasm.

Ⓜ FOR HIM

Move from stroking and caressing her genitals, and start stimulating the perineum (the smooth area between her anus and vagina). Stroke first, then use three fingers and massage firmly.

Let your fingers brush across her anus and see how she reacts. If she pulls away, or clenches her buttocks together, she's either not interested or nervous. If you haven't discussed what you want to do before now, you're playing with fire if you proceed any further!

If she lifts her bottom or presses against

your hand, that's a pretty good indication that she'd like you to continue. Before you do, you *must* apply some lubricant to your finger and her anus. Continue stroking the opening until she's relaxed, then insert the tip of a finger into her rectum. Hold still for a moment or two, then try circling or moving your finger gently in and out. Keep the heel of your hand pressed on the perineum.

Ask her if she's enjoying it before pushing your finger farther inside. If you stimulate her clitoris at the same time, she'll get double the pleasure.

F FOR HER

If his erection's a little halfhearted, this can firm him up in no time. Apply the same techniques listed above on him then . . .

Finger massage his entire rectum, moving in slow circles. Then insert one or two *well-lubricated* fingers about two inches into his rectum. Hold them still until he relaxes, then feel the front wall of the rectum until you find a firm, walnut-sized mass. That's his prostate gland and G-spot. Stroke or press it with a downward movement, using the heel of your hand to press behind the scrotum for extra *uuummmm*.

Ⓜ Ⓕ FOR BOTH OF YOU

If you can't have sex (don't have a condom on you, don't want to have intercourse during your period) or simply want to try something new, give gluteal sex a go. This simply means him using the valley created by her buttock cheeks as an alternative "vagina." It's different, quite exciting, and dead easy. She clenches her buttocks together and rotates her pelvis; he thrusts between them.

A QUICK FIX

If you don't have time for a prolonged sex session or don't particularly want one, give in to the oh-so-sweet pleasures of a "quickie." A quickie is fast, hasty sex of any form. Done at the right time with the right partner, it can be equally, if not more, satisfying than those long, drawn-out sex sessions. The trick is both of you being in the same gloriously turned-on mood simultaneously. This is one instance where you can forget everything I've told you about spending time on foreplay. The whole appeal of a quickie is that it happens spontaneously and the only foreplay you need is "Let's do it." Just remember one thing: a quickie quickly turns from erotically exotic to furiously frustrating if it's the way you have sex *every* time.

A quickie works best:

- When you're both semiclothed. If you're prepared to take your clothes off, you're not impatient enough to enjoy one. *Ripping* them off is a different story.
- When it's spontaneous. Both of you have a sudden urge at the same time.
- When you're both working hard, are too tired for extended sex sessions, but want to keep the fires hot.
- When the female initiates it. Men often feel like fast sex, so he'll be *excruciatingly* turned on if you're the one to suggest it.
- If your sex life is dull and needs an instant lift.

- If one or both of you are a little anxious that you're not performing up to par. It takes the pressure off and lets animal instinct take over.

- When you're *dying* to have sex but you're in public and can't justify disappearing for ages. You're in a park where families are playing ball not so far away? If you've got a short skirt on, pull your panties to one side, sit on his lap (he can unzip under the cover of your skirt), and give him a loving kiss.

"My boyfriend and I were out to dinner with some friends. I went to the toilet, he followed me, and we both thought 'quickie' at the same time. We opened a side door and found an area where the rubbish bins were kept. We had the best sex but it was over in minutes and I figured no one could possibly suspect what we were up to. When I came back to the table, all my friends were killing themselves laughing. They pointed out the window—which had a wonderful view of the rubbish bins below."
Tracy, 29, public relations

The people at the next picnic table will think you're wonderfully romantic!

Some more "quick advice":

- Try doing it in a chair—even better, his or your office chair when no one else is around (don't even think about it if there's a chance of anyone interrupting—it's not worth losing a job or reputation over). You lie back in the chair, he kneels in front of you. Wrap your legs around his bottom.

- Don't restrict quickies to intercourse. Give her oral sex as she's about to walk out the door to meet a girlfriend (leave her clothes on, just pull her knickers to one side); give him the best fellatio he's had in the same situation.

- Start wearing stockings and garters rather than panty hose. They look sexier and allow faster, easier access for quickies.

- Rear-entry positions require minimal undressing. You standing up, facing him, against a wall is another alternative (if your heights match up okay). Stand on one leg and hook the other around him for balance and deeper penetration.

- Give into that *melting* desire, even if you are both dressed to go out and your friends are waiting patiently at a bar. Quickies are quick: you could have *done* it in the two minutes you spent hesitating, one hand on the doorknob.

> **ℹ** *Find sex a bit of a giggle? It's perfectly normal. The sudden release of emotion and tension during or after orgasm can make us laugh. It's all part of the sexual response.*

- Try elevators, the beach, parks, planes, trains, or automobiles. The venue possibilities are endless!

THE RADICAL NEW WAY TO HAVE INTERCOURSE

The coital-alignment technique (CAT) is the brainchild of American psychotherapist Edward Eichel and it's an entirely new approach to intercourse. Even the most jaded sex therapist sat up and took notice when Eichel published his findings back in the early 1990s because they were so astounding. Not only did CAT increase the chance of intercourse orgasms for women, he wrote, it upped the odds of experiencing *simultaneous* orgasms. (Despite common perception, the chances of both of you screaming "Yes! Yes!" at exactly the same time during intercourse are rare—that is unless one of you is faking.)

Eichel tested his theory on forty-three men and women. Before using his technique, 23 percent of the females said they orgasmed during intercourse; this jumped to 77 percent after using CAT. Not one woman had had a simultaneous orgasm with her partner; more than one-third did after using the technique.

The theory behind it is quite simple. Eichel is of the school that believes clitoral stimulation is necessary for women to orgasm. He decided the in-out motion of thrusting was pathetically hopeless at achieving this and invented an alternative "rocking-and-rolling" motion. CAT puts rhythmic pressure on the clitoris and keeps it there. Trouble is, it's not an easy technique for couples to master. You have to think very much "outside the box" to stop doing something that's become second nature after years, so while some devotees now don't have intercourse any other way, most go back to the old in-out-in-out simply because it's easier. Want to give it a try? Here's how to do it . . .

The position
He gets on top of you, lining up his pelvis over yours. His penis is inside you but he's riding "high" so the shaft of it is outside the vagina and pressing against your mons pubis (the fleshy mound covered with pubic hair). He rests his full weight on you and doesn't prop himself up on his elbows. His weight makes him slide forward, toward your shoulders and head. Make sure he doesn't slide back; his pelvis shouldn't slip below yours. Wrap your legs around his thighs and rest your ankles on his calves.

The movement
You're using your pelvis, not your legs and arms, to move. This is the moment you regret

not enrolling in those Arthur Murray dance classes because coordination is everything. The aim is to establish an identical rhythm—both of you moving in exactly the same way at exactly the same speed.

The woman leads in the *upward* stroke: push up and forward to force his pelvis backward. He allows his pelvis to move back but continues to press against yours. The penis disappears into the vagina during the upward stroke. For the *downward* stroke, reverse the process. He forces your pelvis backward and downward. You press against him as he's doing it, pressing your clitoris against the base of his penis. During the downward stroke, his penis rocks forward and presses against the mons pubis, sliding into a shallower position inside the vagina. You're using pressure and counter-pressure, not thrusting in and out.

To orgasm

Instead of speeding up, as most couples do during thrusting, the idea here is to maintain a steady, even pace. Don't speed up, don't slow down. If you've got it right, orgasm will happen naturally—for both of you.

Dear Diary, I had sex today and it was . . .

Maria

Maria, 40, has been married to Ian, 39, for a year. She lives in Brisbane and works as a receptionist at a large community health center. She is highly sexed and frustrated at her husband's lack of interest. She has just started having an affair with a married friend of theirs.

Week one

Had coffee with a girlfriend and we started talking about sex. I was going through one of my horny-as-hell times and trying to explain to her what it felt like. I told her I'm attracted to lots and lots of different kinds of men—often the main attraction is simply that they're new and I haven't conquered them yet. Unless a guy's really unattractive, I can usually find something about him that makes me want him. He might look at me in a way that I know means he wants to sleep with me and that's enough to get the juices flowing. Sometimes, I'll look at his hands and imagine them dipping in and out of me. Once, I was at a barbecue and there was a guy there who was a complete jerk but he had the best body. At one stage, he took off his shirt to show us a scar and he had these fabulous back muscles and brown, gorgeous skin. I felt hot and flushed and if I could have, would have had him there and then. I think I've got more male hormones than female because men understand my feelings about sex totally. (Well, apart from my husband.) When I talk about sex to women they look at me like I'm crazy. But then, most of them don't like sex. I rarely act on my fantasies—though I would if I could get away with it.

Had another erotic dream last night about an old boyfriend. I often have dreams about guys I've dumped who want me back again. In my dreams, I'm sneaking around corners to see them, go back, then get bored again. I'm not that different in real life—once the game is over, I leave. I should never have gotten married because I miss the chase so much. When you're in the middle of someone pursuing you, you're so aware of your body, it feels like it's on fire. I'm like a dog in heat and if the person I'm lusting after comes near me, my body involuntarily arches toward them. That's what I miss about being married. I'm not supposed to have those thoughts anymore, I have to put a tight rein on my natural feelings.

It's funny how when Ian and I have had sex for a few nights running, it's assumed we won't do it for the next three. I looked over at him last night, all tucked in, peacefully asleep, and I wondered if he really cared whether I was satisfied after sex or only interested in getting his own rocks off. Sex with Ian is fine, but that's the problem—it's just so totally, predictably, bloody okay.

Week two

It's now been five days since I last had sex. I've masturbated a billion times but feel like "the real thing," not just me and a copy of Nancy Friday. Went to a party last night and flirted with Gary, this really old friend of ours. He's good-looking and always eyes me up and I think it's obvious we're both attracted to each other. Neither Ian or Gary's wife seem to notice, which is typical: if you're not in tune with sex, I guess you don't pick up vibes between other people either. I bet Gary would be more open to new things than Ian is. I heard a story once that he got caught fucking his secretary in the toilets at work. His wife was devastated but I was turned on. Anyone who screws someone in the toilets is into sex big time. Gary got married really young and his wife is now pregnant. I feel sorry for him. If I get that bored with Ian I can leave. He can't.

From my conversations with other people it seems to me that everyone is bored with their sex life. It's because we're all trying to be monogamous. The other day someone was saying how amazing it was that the boyfriend of this famous celebrity was caught playing around with another woman who wasn't half as attractive. I don't think it's amazing at all. Looks don't come into it: he just wanted someone new. Someone whose every move he didn't know by heart.

I don't believe in PMS because I don't get it,

but I do believe in biorhythms. Sometimes, I can imagine being faithful to Ian, other times it seems impossible. It's a Jekyll and Hyde thing. Reading what I've written so far now seems alien to me because I'm going through a happy-to-be-married period. Today I feel righteous and in love with Ian. We even talked about having kids. All I want to do is have slow, gentle sex with him. What a loony I am!

Week three

I'm still in my "couldn't care less if I never got it again" mood. Had sex on Friday night but it was really frustrating because Ian was giving me oral sex and I was just about to come, then he did something and the delicious bit of the orgasm went and I was just left with the mechanics of it, the contractions minus the pleasure. I told Ian and he said male orgasms are always like that, that the intense, pleasurable bit lasts less than a second. Men are even more stupid than I thought. If their orgasm is so short, why are they in such a hurry to get to it? Why aren't they more into foreplay?

Ian was away on business for two days but the "unsexy" period is coming to a close. I can feel the first stirrings of lust slowly uncoiling in my belly. It sounds dramatic but that's what it feels like. Sometimes I feel controlled by my body because desire takes over and I do things I regret later. It's like this big monster is about to take over my life again—the sheer force of my sexual urges frighten me. I really do love Ian but at those moments, I'd risk it all just to satisfy them.

Week four

I feel really nervous committing this to paper. Remember Gary? The very-very-married-with-pregnant-wife guy I fancied? Well, I slept with him. Ian and I were round at their house on Sunday and we were all slipping into the champagne and swimming in their pool. Ian went off to the liquor store to buy some booze and take-out and the minute he left, Gary's wife said she wanted to pop over and see a friend who was sick. I mean, they asked for it! I felt quite embarrassed at first because it was just Gary and me in the pool. But we started chatting and flirting and next thing, he kissed me. A long, sexy, erotic French kiss. I think I knew it was coming but I was still startled. I laughingly tried to stop him but he kept kissing my neck and it was getting dark and I got so hot I didn't care anymore. He slipped his fingers inside my swimsuit and I was gone. Next minute we were frantically fucking on the side of the pool—and I mean *fucking*—and I climaxed in about one minute flat. I got up quickly afterward and was drying myself off when poor Ian came back, laden with booze, food, and cigarettes. I felt guilty and sad. I've now betrayed him in reality, not just in my head.

Gary called me at work today and said he was sorry. I didn't want him to be sorry, I wanted more and I told him so. I still feel guilty but now that I've thought about it, I've decided to see Gary again. Ian knows I need more from our sex life than he's giving me and yet he still doesn't make an effort. If he's not going to satisfy me, he can't expect me to be faithful. I feel bad about Gary's wife but she's never been a huge fan of mine anyway and I'm not taking him away from her permanently, just borrowing him for a few hours now and again.

My sex life is . . . Guilt-ridden. On one hand, sex gives me the very best moments of my life and I couldn't live without it; on the other, my urges get me in a lot of trouble—like the situation I'm in now. I do love Ian and would like to make it work but the "bad girl" so often beats the "good girl" side of me. I also feel resentful that we've slipped into "married sex" even though we've only been married for a year. I have no idea what will happen now that I'm having an affair but at least Gary's good in bed. Actually, it's not Gary, it's the forbidden part that appeals. In terms of technique, Ian's better.

4

Hot Spots

••

A group of scientists once electronically wired up a mouse so every time it pressed a lever, it triggered an orgasm. The mouse died within twenty-four hours—from orgasm over-dose. While the researchers were tucked up in their beds, he was pressing that lever, over and over and over again until his little body could take no more. That's what I call dying with a smile on your face.

While I certainly don't think orgasm should ever be the ultimate aim of any sex session (you're both human and one or both probably won't climax every single time), it's always rather nice if you do have one. Which is the point of this chapter. I hope these suggestions will make your orgasms even more delicious than they are already.

FOREPLAY FOR FAMILIAR LOVERS

Think back to when you met each other. The first few dates—particularly the ones before you've had intercourse—are one, long, deliciously exciting foreplay session. Remember getting an erection by simply watching her walk across a room? Being told off by your friends for snogging him in hallways at parties? People chastising you for not being able to keep your hands off each other? This is what we're aiming to recapture. Sadly, that initial sell-your-mother-to-get-it type of lust that characterizes new relationships disappears all too quickly and sex gets relegated to a certain time slot and place.

Sometimes this is

> **Who has the best sex—stay-at-home-and-watch-television couples or those who party the night away? Studies prove those who stay in have better sex, more often.**

not only sensible but necessary. If you've just started a new job, the last thing you're thinking about is whether the knickers you put on that morning are sexy enough for him to peel off that night. If he's struggling with family problems, chances are he's not going to surprise you with a Chippendales-style strip before the six o'clock news. But the rest of the time—when you're simply coping with the usual hiccups of routine, run-of-the-mill life—give sex the priority it deserves.

Memorize the next three sentences. Our most erogenous zone is the brain. The most erotic tool you have at your disposal is your imagination. The biggest turn-on of all is anticipation. Repeat them one more time. Learn how to combine the three and *wham!*, you've just raised your sex life from ho-hum to hellishly horny. Most of us think of foreplay as genital touching and oral sex. Wrong. Foreplay can start at six o'clock in the morning, continue while you're both at work, be drawn out through dinner, then, when you're both *begging* to touch each other, the physical part starts.

Skeptical that anyone actually *does* the things I'm suggesting? You're dead right. Few people do—that's why everyone's madly bonking everyone else behind each other's backs. It's easy to pick the couples who put effort into their sex lives. They're the two sixty-year-olds next door who hold hands when they're out perusing the roses. That devilish gleam in their eyes isn't put there from bingo. Ditto the couple you've always envied because sexual sparks seem to *fly* between them, yet they've been together five years. Here's how they do it . . .

- **Combine romance with eroticism.** You feel great when he sends you flowers, why not return the favor? If you think they aren't quite his style, then try sending a bottle of expensive vintage champagne, red wine, or port. Now turn that loving gesture into a sexy one. Enclose a note explaining in great detail exactly what he did to deserve such luxurious spoils. (No, not washing your car—the to-die-for oral

The most popular places to have sex outside the bedroom? The car, the beach, in a swimming pool.

sex he gave you last week. Got it?) Your postscript details what you're aching for him to do to you that night!

- **Become a bookworm.** Invest $100 in your love life by walking into any good bookshop and walking out with an armful of sex books. You've already bought this one, now branch out into areas that particularly tickle your fancy: tantric sex, fantasies, how to have a dozen orgasms an hour. You don't have to read them cover to cover, just dip inside once in a while to keep things fresh and imaginative. While you're there, splash out on a racy, erotic novel. Find the good bits and read them out to each other as a form of foreplay.

- **For the confident.** Use your vaginal juices as perfume. Yup, I'm not kidding. Slip your finger inside, then touch it around your throat, your breasts, on your lips. He won't know what it is but he won't be able to keep his hands off you.

- **Have a bed picnic.** Set up chilled wine and an ice bucket, foods you can eat with your

fingers (fresh fruit, chocolates); have an
erotic movie playing in the background on
the bedroom VCR.

- **Once isn't always enough.** There's a lot of
hype about women having more than one
orgasm but he likes double helpings, too.
Have sex in the morning on the weekend,
then drag him back to bed an hour later.
- **Get wet.** Water does wonderful things: it
makes us weightless and flexible and ensures
every part of both of you tastes and smells
wonderful. While I wouldn't recommend
having intercourse in water (it dries up
lubrication and forcing water up the vagina
isn't recommended), the bath, a spa, a
swimming pool, or the sea are great places
to start off.
- **Be her sex slave for a day.** An especially
good idea if you're broke and her birthday
is looming. All you need to do is offer to
devote one entire day to pleasuring her. She
gets to order you around unashamedly—
and whether it's serving her an erotic break-
fast in bed, feeding her grapes and

strawberries Roman-style, or spending the day dressed only in your Calvins, you're not allowed to utter even a *word* of complaint.

- **Take a tip from the old classic *The Story of O.*** The character in the novel is taught not to give all of herself each time she makes love. Use the same philosophy and instead of each sex session running the gauntlet from kissing to intercourse, concentrate on one activity at a time: kissing and fondling-only sessions (no tongues, no penises, just fingers), oral sex without intercourse, and intercourse without oral sex.

- **Flirt with each other**—even if you've been together years! Experts say flirting sends natural amphetamines and endorphins surging through the body, stimulating an instant emotional high not unlike orgasm. Pretend you've just met him and act as you did at the beginning. Dress sexily, look him dead in the eye when he's talking, twirl your hair around a finger. Be

Love hurts: 44 percent of men and 41 percent of women like getting love bites.

aware of your body when you move in front of him and chances are he'll sit up and take notice, too.

- **Send sexy notes.** The written word is extremely powerful. Plant notes everywhere (preferably not just before her mother comes to visit). In the fridge stuck to the fruit juice, in her briefcase and makeup bag. Each one describes bits of her you find *sooo* sexy. The next time, make them ten things you'd love to do to her right that second.

- **Tease.** You've got friends over for dinner? Smack him up against the fridge, cup his penis with your hand, and give him a huge kiss while he's helping you in the kitchen. Chatter innocently away to your guests while he hides out there, waiting for his erection to go down.

- **Go out without panties on.** This is one steamy idea even the least courageous of females can pull off. All you need to do is dress up for an evening out—and forget to put on your panties. You can either tell him about it, or "accidentally" show him by crossing your legs Sharon Stone–style.

- **Feeling a little bored at her next staff get-together?** Make things infinitely more interesting by feigning sickness, then take her with you to the bathroom. Emerge later feeling much better, thank you.

- **Be a voyeur.** Madonna's done it. So can you. We're talking mirrors and using them as sex props. Madonna crawled and masturbated above a mirror laid flat on

the floor. If yours is on the wardrobe door, it's pretty difficult to follow her lead.

"God knows what it was, but about three months ago, I went through a stage where all I could think about was sex. A lot of the time, I kept my mouth shut because we'd be over at Ian's mother's house or something. Then I started telling him about it and it built the sexual tension wonderfully. I rang him at work one day and told him I was masturbating and he canceled a meeting, drove home, and we had the best sex ever. It hasn't been this good since the beginning."
Helen, 32, mother

Instead, try making love in front of any available mirror in the house (angled so you can see her rather than vice versa if she's shy).

- **Be his mistress.** If he's going to have an affair, make sure it's with you. Arrange to meet him at lunchtime in the bar of a plain but presentable hotel. Book a room, buy a bottle of champagne, and have forbidden, illicit, wild sex.

- **Get into the mood beforehand.** Masturbate several times during the day while you think about what the two of you will get up to that night—preferably telling her exactly what you're doing over the phone as you're doing it. Stop short of an orgasm, unless you're a premature ejaculator. If you are, masturbate an hour before you have sex— you'll last longer.

- **Remember kissing?** It's what you used to do when you first met. Many couples find that kissing stops once the relationship gets going or dwindles to a quick snog before getting down to business. A long, passionate kiss can do more to turn both of you on than putting your hands straight down the front of his trousers. It's more intimate than intercourse (which is why many sex workers won't do it).

- **Have intercourse with your clothes on.** Feel each other through your clothing, put your leg in between her thighs and let her gyrate against it.
- **Be pushy.** Bearing down with your vaginal muscles during intercourse seems to trigger orgasm for many women.
- **Keep your eyes open.** Watch what's going on when you have sex, look into their face, watch your genitals moving in and out. Stimulate the sense of sight, not just touch.
- **Be unpredictable.** Let's face it—you're hardly going to widen his eyes with astonishment if you suggest having sex on a Saturday night as you both climb into bed. But you will catch him unawares if you cuddle him from behind when he's washing the car, washing up, or reading a book. Start fondling him, bring him to the brink of

Great Timing . . .
When's the best
time to have sex?
In the morning.
His testosterone levels
peak around 9 A.M. and
if you've been
together a while, your
cycle probably echoes
his. An orgasm?
Midway through your
menstrual cycle.
You're twice as likely
to orgasm because
your nerve endings are
at their most sensitive.

orgasm, then refuse to follow through until later.

- **Bare all.** For a truly original Valentine's Day gift, shave your pubic hair into the shape of a heart or shave it off completely. The sight of your totally exposed genitals will make him jump to attention!

- **Turn her on in the most inappropriate places.** This is a tricky one. Done at the right time, it works fantastically, but it does have a tendency to backfire. Many sex books advise you whisper suggestive somethings into her ear while you're out to dinner with her boss, for instance. Sounds fabulously erotic, but in practice her boss is likely to think you're horribly rude, or that he has something stuck between his teeth and you're making fun of him. Ditto the ringing him at work bit. You want to get him hot and bothered but not so flustered he ends up blowing the deal of the century. By all means try it—just scope out the situation before you launch into your spiel.

- **Be anonymous.** Remember those silly masks you bought for the dress-up affair you both went to? Dig them out, put them on, laugh yourself stupid for five minutes, then have sex. Let your fantasies run wild and pretend you don't know each other.

- **Wake her up with the ultimate greeting**—licking her vagina. Do the same for him by licking his penis.

- **Make the move.** If your partner is always the one to initiate sex, the message you're sending is this: I do it to please you, not because I want to. This leaves both of you feeling cheated. The person who initiates sex feels sexier because they're taking control and giving themselves power. Surely you've watched enough movies by now to know that power's one of the biggest sexual turn-ons there is. Be the boss by suggesting sex and taking the lead role during love-making as well. Let them lie back while you do *all* the work.

- **Lie a little.** He's away on business? The next time he calls you late at night, skip the what-did-you-do-today stuff and tell him, in intimate detail, what you're wearing. No, not the truth—that scruffy old T-shirt and thick white socks are silky, black French panties and a camisole. Move onto what you're going to do to him the minute you get your hands on him. The juicier and more explicit the better.

> Q: What are most couples doing at 10:34 P.M.?
> A: Making love. That's the average time researchers came up with when they asked 198 couples when they had sex.

- **Slide around on satin sheets.** So kitsch they're almost fashionable, you can't help but feel sensual with satin against bare skin. Great sex comes from indulging *all* the senses and satin sheets are one of a million ways to do it.

Appeal to and vary one sense each time you make love and you'll never be bored again. Use music to stimulate his sense of hearing; talk to her while you're having sex, giving a blow-by-blow description of how she's making you feel. Ignite his sense of smell by burning oils, wearing perfume, or letting him enjoy the naturally sweet scent your body emits when you're aroused. Touch is stimulated by different textures: use your hair, feathers, and scarves, as well as fingertips. Use food, champagne, and all of your body parts to excite his taste buds.

- **Plan a dirty weekend.** More than one lackluster sex life has been saved by a spicy weekend

> "I've been married nine years but I could watch Sally undress for bed a million times and never be bored. She's always so distracted, she doesn't notice me watching, but I love her breasts and the way she always fluffs her hair up and pouts in the mirror when she's naked . . . even if the only thing she's craving is sleep."
> Calvin, 43, architect

bounding about on a king-size bed. Book the best hotel you can afford, pick her up from work on Friday night, and disappear into the sunset for a weekend she won't forget in a hurry.

- **Dress for success.** He adores red lipstick, black stockings, and high heels? You've got no excuse—any little black number suits this treatment. Make a night of it by playing the vamp, playing with your hair, playing with him under the table. She melts when you walk around the house in nothing but a pair of blue jeans, top button of the fly temptingly undone? Unless it's below freezing temperatures, indulge her on weekends.

- **Make a pact to try one new thing each fortnight.** If you're too shy to launch into my other suggestions, start off simple. Have a bath together, give each other a foot massage, take off her top or his shirt without using your hands. Once you feel more comfortable, you can move into things like making love to them with their hands tied behind their back and (the real biggie) masturbating in front of each other. Get him to lick your fingers while you're masturbating yourself—you'll feel less embarrassed and both of you will find it a turn-on.

- **Turn undressing for bed into an art form.** It doesn't matter what you're wearing, it's how you take it off that counts. Unbutton tops slowly, stretch luxuriously as you pull that sweater over your head, put one leg up on the bed as you roll down your panty hose. When you're naked, admire yourself for a minute in the mirror, running your hands over your breasts and hips. Not only will it keep him focused on your body and remove the familiarity of seeing you naked, it helps create a positive body image.

- **Suck each of his fingers as though it were a small**

> **❓ What do most women do straight after sex?**
> 43 percent have a shower
> 20 percent clean their teeth
> 30 percent roll over and go to sleep
> 7 percent have a cigarette

penis. Circle your tongue lazily around her palm to simulate oral sex.

- **Learn to love oral sex.** Don't just do it to please him or her, revel in it. Crave it, concentrate, make noises to show you're enjoying it as much as they are. Switch from intercourse to oral sex and back again for sensational contrasts.
- **If you're excited, show it.** The biggest turn-on of all is seeing how much you're exciting your partner. If he's driving you wild, show him—better still, say so.

Enough already! In the midst of all this lust, it's worth pointing out that no one can be a sexual dynamo all the time. If you don't feel like having sex, say so, and let him do the same. That way, it's guilt-free on both sides and it will save either of you putting on lukewarm performances.

How to Find Your G-Spot

Ernst Grafenberg started all the fuss in Germany in 1944. He published a paper claiming there was an area in the upper wall of the vagina so erotically charged that a woman was guaranteed to orgasm if it was stimulated. Fellow researchers pooh-poohed the idea, so Grafenberg closed his mouth and kept it shut. About four decades later, a team of American psychologists also argued that women could have multiple orgasms, without clitoral stimulation, if the same area was stimulated. Again, the idea met with little support.

Since then, modern science has proved that our vaginal walls are pleasurably sensitive and there seems little doubt that there is definitely a "hidden area" that produces intense excitement when aroused in *some* women. But not all females have one. (The male G-spot is less controversial: it was identified almost immediately as the prostate gland.)

So, for women, the debate still rages. Most sex therapists are convinced that it does exist, but a few fix you with a "not that old myth" withering stare if you even mention it. Still, worth launching an expedition to find out, don't you think? So here goes . . .

Finding hers

The G-spot is a small cluster of nerve endings and glands near the woman's urethra or urinary tract. Because it only swells and stands out from the vaginal wall when aroused, the G-spot usually can't be felt unless it's stimulated.

The easiest way to find it yourself is to squat—maybe even sit on the toilet. Now, insert a finger into your well-lubricated vagina, curving it so you're hitting the front wall (imagine you're aiming toward your belly). Feel around a little, hopefully causing the G-spot to swell so you can pinpoint it, until you find a raised area that feels textured. Most experts say it's around the size of a large pea.

Some women find their first stimulation

"When I first went out with Scott, he was always fiddling around inside me and I thought 'What's he doing?' The third time we made love, I found out he was looking for my G-spot. And he found it. I can't orgasm from that alone, but if he has one hand stimulating that and the other on my clitoris, I'm putty."
Marie, 20, secretary

of the G-spot distinctly uncomfortable. It can produce similar feelings to wanting to pee. Empty your bladder first or sit on the toilet when you first try. If you relax into the sensation, the feeling will pass.

Hold your finger still to begin with, then experiment. Don't press hard and constantly— a gentle, stroking motion is better. Try stroking left to right and back again or in circles; in other words, so your fingers are *passing over* the G-spot without concentrating on it directly. G-spot orgasms feel different from clitoral orgasms. If you have one, you may find you ejaculate a small amount of clear fluid (which isn't urine, by the way).

It's best if you lie on a bed, with pillows underneath your bottom, for your partner to find it. It makes the area more easily accessible for him to follow the instructions. Once found, he can combine G-spot stimulation with oral sex or while he's masturbating you. The best intercourse positions to hit the spot are woman-on-top or him behind (doggie-style).

Finding his

Just because you haven't found yours, doesn't mean you shouldn't try to find his (it might even give you some clues).

Like the female G-spot, the male's is situated near the urethra. Unlike ours, his has a medical name—the prostate gland—and it has an organic function. There's another point of difference: while we can find our own, it's rather difficult for him to stimulate his because it's up his rectum. He can try (by lying on his back, knees bent and feet flat on the floor or knees drawn up to his chest, inserting his thumb and pressing against the front wall), but it's simpler if you find it for him.

Apply some personal lubricant to your finger (nails trimmed and clean) and get him to lie on his back. Gently insert the finger into his anus, then feel up the front rectal wall until you find something that feels like a walnut. Hold your finger still until he's relaxed, then start massaging firmly in a downward direction. He can draw his knees up to his chest once you've found it.

It can take a little while for him to orgasm (so make sure you're both comfortable) but it's worth the effort. If it works, you'll be in the unique position of having given him an orgasm without even touching his penis! Male fans claim not only are G-spot orgasms more intense, they ejaculate in a continuous stream rather than in spurts.

Once you're an expert, try massaging his G-spot while you're giving him oral sex, or stimulate it during him-on-top intercourse positions.

One note about hygiene: always wash your hands after inserting fingers into rectums. If you touch your own genitals you can inadvertently transfer bacteria into your vagina.

DEEPER, LONGER, BETTER, MORE . . .

Up the number and intensity of your orgasms by trying any (and all) of the following.

- **Don't race to get to the finish line.** The longer you've spent on foreplay, the more enhanced it will be for both of you.
- **Slow his down, speed yours up.** You envy the fact that he can orgasm with one hand

behind his back (literally); he's jealous of your ability to hover in the oh-Jesus-John-I'm-just-about-there stage for ages. Anything that delays his orgasm will increase his enjoyment; anything that makes her more easily orgasmic will increase her pleasure potential.

- **Teach him control.** As you're stimulating him, get him to tell you how he's feeling by rating it on a scale of one to ten (ten being the can't-go-back-now point). Drive him to distraction by revving him up to a seven or eight, then slowing it down again, several times over, before letting him go all the way.
- **Alternate oral sex with intercourse.** If he's too close to coming, change activities. Get him to give you oral sex until he feels more in control.
- **Touch his penis frequently.** The more often your hand, tongue, or vagina touches it, the less sensitive he'll be and the longer he'll last.

- **Don't be a clock-watcher.** Stop wondering whether his tongue's gone numb or if he'll miss the football game if you don't come soon. The best lover in the world is the man who says, "Take your time, honey—I love doing it to you as much as you like receiving it" (and means it). You can't fight biology; both of you should accept that it's more complicated for you to have an orgasm than him.

- **Give her a head start.** Give her an orgasm through oral sex or masturbation *before* intercourse. Give him one orally, so his second intercourse orgasm lasts longer.

- **Don't try too hard and don't freak if you don't have one.** Remember when you were a kid and tried to touch a rainbow? Orgasms can be just as elusive. Reach just a little higher, you think, and you'll have one, but the next minute it's slipped through your (or his) fingers. Lots of women move steadily toward the point of having an orgasm then, out of nowhere, something intrudes. *I forgot Jane's birthday last week,* you think, or you hear your flatmate's key in the door or remember you have to confront your boss in the morning. Your orgasm potential's disappeared, not forever, but certainly for that session. The same thing can happen if he changes technique or rhythm at the wrong time; everything that has built up fades away. Trying harder will only make things worse. Instead, accept that you will have one next time you make love (making sure it's sooner rather than later) and you will. Stress out about it, start tormenting yourself with thoughts like "That's it. This is going to happen every time and I'll never have one" and you'll set up more psychological roadblocks than the average detour.

- **Masturbate with him rather than alone.** If you don't have an orgasm during intercourse, give yourself one afterward. He can watch or place his hand over yours.

- **Don't treat her clitoris like it's a lift button.** Some men think the more they press it, the quicker you'll zoom to the top. (Doesn't work for lifts, either.) Most women climax if you work around the base of the clitoris rather than touch it directly.

Orgasms promote cardiovascular conditioning, make the skin glow, improve overall body tone, and can cure menstrual cramps. The emotional release makes us feel less irritable and more relaxed.

- **Prime yourself for sex by turning yourself on beforehand.** When he's talking to friends, think about what that tongue will do to you later, how much better his fingers would feel inside you rather than wrapped around a beer glass.
- **Stop worrying about what you look like.** If your partner isn't someone you can let go with, without fear of criticism, they're not the right choice. In, or out of, the bedroom.
- **Show each other how to do it.** Not like an army commander where you're shouting "Left" and "Right" but "Hmmm, that feels fantastic when you do it really slow," or "God, that's great. Do it harder."

- **Masturbate more.** Researchers claim it increases your sexual appetite because the more sex we have, the more our bodies expect.
- **Make noise.** It sounds and feels sexy.
- **Get wet.** It doesn't mean you're not turned on if you're not lubricating like crazy; you might just be at a different stage of the menstrual cycle, stressed, or tired. Accept that sometimes you'll need to add artificial lubricant like K-Y.
- **Both do Kegel exercises.** Women do them to tighten their vagina and give them more control over orgasm; men can use the same genital workout to orgasm more frequently. Simply squeeze and hold the same muscle that stops you peeing when there's not a bathroom in sight. It's called the "PC" muscle. The experts maintain male masters of Kegels can become "multiorgasmic." He can try contracting his PC muscle hard, for five seconds, as he's hovering on the brink of orgasm. Reputedly, this delays ejaculation but he'll "feel" an orgasm in his brain.

Potentially, he could climax several times before having an ejaculatory orgasm.

- **Give him a squeeze.** Squeezing the base of the penis firmly for a few seconds can delay ejaculation.
- **Fantasize guilt-free.** Many women and men use fantasy to launch themselves into orgasmic orbit; some can't achieve one without it. Quit the guilt trip. Your partner can't read minds, remember?

THE KNOCK-THEIR-SOCKS-OFF EROTIC GENITAL MASSAGE

Genital massage has been around for thousands of years, but has only recently been discovered by Western society—and westernized, of course! The true, unadulterated version draws heavily on the Kama Sutra and tantric sex and is preceded by all sorts of bizarre, complicated rituals. But for our purposes (and because, to be honest, I've never found things like breathing in each other's breath terribly sexy), we'll skip straight to the nitty-gritty. You'll have a bit of a giggle over the names, but these explicit techniques are easy to learn and can transform the most mediocre lover into a wow-honey-that-was-*incredible* sort overnight. You may need to have the book beside you the first couple of times to follow the instructions, but when you've mastered it . . . well, your lovers won't forget you in a hurry!

❺ FOR HER

Most men assume the "power position" during sex, so erotic massage will be especially pleasurable for him because it's a totally different sensation. Instead of you lying back and him doing all the work, he gets to relax and experience the sensation of touch while *you* take control.

Most of these techniques work best with him lying on his back on the bed, legs comfortably apart, and you kneeling between them. You'll need lots of oil; a water-based

> *Average time two-thirds of couples spend on foreplay: between six and twenty minutes. Number of men who agree it's possible to have a satisfying sex life without penile penetration: 43 percent.*

one, sold at most sex shops, is ideal but unscented massage oil or baby oil will do the trick. Ask him to give you feedback all the way through the massage, saying which strokes and pressure he prefers. Watch his face and read his body language for clues. The idea isn't for him to orgasm quickly but to immerse himself in the concept of receiving pleasure. If it seems like he's losing control, stop what you're doing and lay both hands on top of his penis. Hold still, maintaining a firm but not heavy pressure, for about thirty seconds to calm him down. If you want him to orgasm, speed up the strokes.

Spiraling the stalk

This is great to use if he's having trouble getting an erection.

Hold the base of the penis with one hand and take a firm hold of it with your other. Start at the bottom and slide to the top using a circular, twisting motion as you wind toward the head. Picture a corkscrew—that's the sort of movement you're imitating.

When you get to the head of the penis, use the

> "My girlfriend puts a hell of an effort into our sex life. Each time we have sex, she'll introduce something new—whether it's a position, a technique, or a location. It used to freak me out. I couldn't help obsessing that she'd done all this with someone else (or was having a bit on the side and picking up tricks that way). Then I figured she just had a vivid imagination and was really into sex. She drives me nuts outside the bedroom, but there's no way I'm letting go of her."
> Neil, 19, mechanic

palm of your hand to caress the entire surface. Only work upward.

The twelve o'clock stroke

Save this one until he's aroused and has a full erection. It's called "twelve o'clock" because you're moving directly upward in a straight line.

Open your hand so your thumb and fingers are separated to make an L-shaped space. Slide your hand underneath the testicles until they rest between that space (if you're using your left hand, your fingers would be on the left-hand side of the testicles, thumb on the right). Push up a little so you're lifting them slightly.

With your palm down, separate the first two fingers of your other hand to make a V and slide the penis between them, working upward from the testicles to the head and tilting your hand so the flat of your hand brushes up against the shaft of the penis. Only work upward with this stroke. When you reach the head, remove your hand and start from the bottom again. Don't just slide up the middle; try sliding up the sides as well.

Making fire
This is the final technique because he's almost certain to orgasm.

Imagine you have a stick between your hands and are trying to start a fire by rolling it. Hold the palms of your hands straight, facing either side of his penis.

Using a rolling/rubbing motion, start at the bottom of his penis and slide upward, then down again, keeping the motion consistent and rhythmic. His penis will sit naturally between your palms. Start slowly, then build pressure and speed when he approaches orgasm.

Ⓜ FOR HIM

Rather than foreplay, think of her erotic massage as a sensual gift. It may lead to intercourse but she's far more likely to enjoy it if there's no pressure to have sex at the end. As with the male massage, most of these techniques work best if she's lying on her back with her legs apart and you're kneeling between them. Put pillows under her knees and let her legs fall open naturally: it's more comfortable and she'll feel less vulnerable and exposed.

Don't use oil on her vagina; use a thin, liquid lubricant. K-Y is too heavy. Try Astroglide, Glyde, Liquid Silk, or Sylk (available at pharmacies and sex shops). Warm the lubricant by rubbing it between your fingers.

Ask her to tell you which strokes feel best, whether she prefers a firm or gentle touch. If you're unsure, err on the too gentle side; she'll probably push against your hand if she wants more pressure. Keep the rhythm regular and don't chop and change techniques too much. Watch her face—if it's relaxed, so is her body.

Remember, erotic massage isn't meant to replace foreplay. Use these techniques every single time you make love and sex will, once more, become routine

In the quest for orgasm, 75 percent of women rate foreplay as more important than intercourse. More than half the male readers of Penthouse say they don't get as much foreplay as they'd like to make their orgasms more intense.

and predictable. Instead, adapt the strokes to suit her individual preferences, combine techniques, invent some of your own—then transport her to orgasmic heaven!

The two-finger stroke

Nicknamed "the bread-and-butter" stroke, this technique is the easiest and simplest way of giving her pleasure.

Rest your thumb and index finger at the top of the vagina (the end where the clitoris is), on the inside lips. Rotate your fingers around the top of the clitoris, then move your fingers downward.

Massage and roll evenly, rubbing up and down on either side of the vagina, settling into an even rhythm.

She's ready for more direct clitoral stimulation when she opens her legs wider, pushes against your hand, or raises her pelvis off the bed.

Rock around the clock

It's extremely useful to imagine a clock dial surrounding the vaginal area, the top (near her pubic hair) being the twelve o'clock position and the lowest point (near the vaginal opening) being six o'clock. If she tells you what feels good, you can memorize the position (three o'clock, nine o'clock) for next time. Plus she can direct you more accurately. This technique was adapted from the tantric original by the outrageous (but ever inventive) sex guru Annie Sprinkle.

Using the tip of your finger, move around the clitoris in a circular motion. Using bigger circles continue the circular motion down the entire length of the vagina, alternating with stroking, teasing, caresses with your fingertips.

Now move back to the clitoris and circle directly over it with a fingertip. Some women don't like direct clitoral stimulation, so check with her which area feels best when stimulated, using the "clock" as a guide.

Try "pulling" the clitoris between two fingers. It's not actually possible to get a grip on it, but the pulling motion feels fabulous!

Entering the garden

This is a double-action stroke that works on the G-spot and clitoris simultaneously to bring most women to orgasm.

Insert a finger (or two) into her well-lubricated vagina, curving them so you're working on the front wall (imagine you're aiming upward to her stomach). Hold your finger still for a few seconds; she may move against it, but don't apply pressure until she feels comfortable.

The G-spot feels like a small, textured lump. When aroused, it engorges with blood and becomes more sensitive. Once you've found it, move into a "come here" motion, like you're beckoning someone with your finger. Don't press hard or constantly; a gentle, beckoning, stroking motion is usually far more pleasurable. Try a zigzag motion so your fingers are passing over the G-spot without concentrating on it too directly.

With your other hand, "rock around the clock," circling the clitoris with your finger, thumb, or a flat-surfaced vibrator. Also try moving directly backward and forward over it as she's about to orgasm.

Dear Diary, I had sex today and it was . . .

Robert
Robert, 35, separated from his wife three years ago. He works as an account executive for a finance firm and describes his sex life as "active but selective."

Week one
I'm making love to Sarah but it's not really Sarah, it's Linda. Linda was a married woman I had an affair with over one year ago but she still haunts me. I met her through a mutual work friend at a

function and we ended up getting drunk together and smooching on the balcony. Her husband was working. She was so beautiful and so unattainable, I thought that was it. But she called me soon after I met her and asked if she could drop in for coffee. So we started meeting and kissing and cuddling, then one day she came over and stripped right down to her underwear before snuggling up to me. I knew she wanted sex but I didn't want to push it. I mean, she was married and on this massive guilt-trip. We had intercourse but it felt like she wouldn't give herself fully although she had no trouble orgasming. I did—I was nervous as hell. For some reason, she didn't want much foreplay. It was like kissing, touching, then *bam*! she wanted penetration. I felt like I was starting halfway through. I'm not the sort of guy who can just drop my duds and get into it. She ended the affair soon after that so we only had intercourse three times. I knew the score. I knew she would end it but I've never forgotten her. I'd love to go out with someone as good-looking as her again and have other guys check out your girl. It's a huge ego boost.

Sarah's probably a better fuck, if truth be told, and she gives a brilliant head job. She's the opposite of Linda: she wants a relationship and gives her all. The first time I slept with Sarah, we had sex with her six-month-old son asleep beside us. I thought it was a bit outrageous but the kid was fast asleep. It didn't turn me on at all—I actually felt quite uncomfortable and couldn't look at the child—but I admired Sarah for going for what she wanted. I'm the guilty one now. Sarah loves me and I love her but I make love to Linda whenever I touch her.

Week two

Sarah's gone away for a week with her folks so I meet some friends down at the local. There's a girl there who's exotic and very horny. We talk and I give her my phone number. She's called Cristina and is from South America. That was on Friday. On Tuesday, she called me at 11:30 P.M., said she was lonely and would I like to come over. I was in bed but she said she was down, so off I went. Cristina lived in a penthouse apartment overlooking the city and her flatmates were out. She answered the door wearing a see-through lace teddy, led me to the couch, pushed me back, and just went for it. Then she led me to the balcony and within five minutes of walking in the door, I was standing there, pants around my ankles, getting a head job while overlooking Sydney Harbour! She took me into her room and she had this mirror that she loved to watch herself in. She wanted it doggie-style and kept on saying, "Fuck me, fuck me like an animal." I felt like I should write in to *Penthouse*. It was like one of those letters you read and never believe. I took her phone number but it was pretty obvious she only got off on someone new. I don't think I ever approach any sex session as just a fuck. I guess I hope they'll all lead to something. I told the guys at the pub what had happened. One of them said, "Mate, that must have been the best sex of your life." I guess it was because it was so unexpected, but the best is always the last one you've had really. I thought my wife gave the best head job, then I thought Linda did, then Sarah. Now Cristina's in front.

Week three

Sarah's back. I expected her to be relaxed, tanned, and keen for sex; instead, she's irritable and worn out because she had a shit time. Sex is awful because she's not responsive. I hate that more than anything. The worst sex I ever had was with a girl who led me from the living room to the bedroom by my penis. She instigated it all and I thought I was in for the ride of my life. But when I penetrated her, she lay there like a dead fish. I don't know if she was terribly pissed and it hit her then or what. She couldn't have been bored because we'd just started! Anyway, it goes down as the absolute worst sex of all and I think it's a worry that sex with Sarah reminded me of it. Sarah wants a commitment but I'm not sure I want to. I'm feeling incredibly pressured and also not sure I want to take on someone else's child. I've already got two of my own.

Week four

Cristina called and Sarah answered the phone. Neither were terribly impressed and even I wouldn't have believed the story I made up to try and get out of it. For some weird reason, Cristina was upset that I hadn't told her about Sarah. A bit much when she had her mouth wrapped around my penis before I'd even had a chance to speak! I feel guilty but pissed off for feeling like that. I've never promised Sarah a monogamous relationship—she just took it for granted—and Cristina was obviously just in it for the sex. My month ends where it started: with fantasies about Linda. Even though she was married, at least I knew where I stood.

My sex life is . . . A hell of a lot more interesting than it was when I was married. My wife was pretty conservative, and missionary was about it. I didn't have much experience before I got married so I'm making up for it now but aiming for quality, not quantity. I find women so much more liberated and in touch with their sexuality than the first time round. Sometimes it freaks me a little bit and I worry I'm not going to be able to satisfy them. I think that's why I'm so into foreplay; I feel more confident with my oral sex skills. Besides, intercourse is intercourse and most women's vaginas feel pretty much the same. There's only one girl who's stood out from the pack and she had a vise for a vagina. Her grip was incredible!

5

Fanning the Flames

·····································

Monogamy and monotony don't have to go together like peaches and cream. Sex really *can* get better as the years roll on. There's just one catch: you have to be prepared to put creativity and effort into your sex life to introduce the variety that's naturally lacking when you're making love to the same body over and over again. I admit it up front: it's an effort at first. If you're mind-numbingly bored by each other's bits, it's a real slog to force interest and try a few new things. But one or two sessions later, it'll seem less like hard work because it works. One month from that, you start to remember how much you used to enjoy sex. Six weeks on you'll start grinning at each other whenever you think about last night. And two months on? Your friends will be calling to say "Where were you two last night? You never seem to go out much anymore . . ."

LIGHTS, CAMERA, ERECTION!: ACTING OUT A SEXUAL FANTASY

That lurid reverie about your primary school teacher and raspberry jelly isn't first-date material. But sharing and acting out some fantasies is an excellent idea if you've been together awhile, talk openly about sex, and, most important, know that your innermost thoughts won't be the subject of your partner's next boys' or girls' night out.

Literally thousands of us secretly use fantasies to orgasm during sex, so owning up and acting them out can be the lustiest sex game you've played in years. Provocative barmaids,

> **Fifty-five percent of men have fantasized about a threesome, compared to 27 percent of women.**

nymphomaniac nurses, dominatrixes and boot-licking boy toys, sexy slave girls and sultans, muscle-bound bikies and straightlaced career women: find the role that appeals to you and make like you're in the movies—though I strongly advise *against* turning it into one. "Of course it's for our eyes only," you both purr in the lovey-dovey stage. It's a different story when you ditch him for his best friend and a copy "accidentally" gets dropped in your mother's postbox.

How do you suggest acting out a fantasy or finding out about theirs? Wait until you're both feeling relaxed and intimate, then say you had an amazingly sexy dream last night. Tell your partner about it and see what reaction you get. If they seem nicely titillated, confess that it's actually been a fantasy of yours for ages, and ask what are some of theirs. Once you're both talking, it's relatively easy to move into a line like, "Hey, I've just had a great idea. Why don't we act them out for a bit of fun?"

Try to choose fantasies that appeal to *both* of

> *Of all our sexual fantasies, bondage (tying each other up) is the one we're most likely to act out. Twenty-three percent of men just fantasize about bondage, 27 percent have done it. Twenty-five percent of women just dream about it, 26 percent take it through to real life.*

you, particularly the first time round, and work out the scenario together beforehand: what you'll each wear, how you want them to act and vice versa. Then use your own imagination to embellish the story, adding a few surprises to the screenplay, maybe taking it even further. You could also try each writing down three favorite fantasies along with instructions on how you'd like to act them out. Write them on separate pieces of paper and put them in a jar for either of you to fish out when you feel like playing. You won't know what fantasy it is until you open it, and neither will they.

Acting out fantasies doesn't have to be literal: symbolism is often all that's needed. Got an anal sex fantasy but don't want to actually do it? Pretend you are while having vaginal sex doggie-style. Use stockings and ties, not rough ropes for tying-up games; and there's no need to tie knots tight—the idea is to fake a struggle rather than to have a real one because your circulation's cut off. Lavishly expensive props aren't necessary (though they are worth thinking about for favorite fantasies): black stockings and high heels turn her into a prostitute; jeans and no shirt (and a suitably subservient expression) turn him into a sex slave.

Remember to set the scene using music and different rooms of the house (take it outside if it would work better) but don't stress about it. You don't have to be too literal—it's the sense of the fantasy that you're re-creating. Similarly, don't be surprised if the first time you do it, either (or both) of you nearly explode from trying to stop the giggles. Laughing together is all part of it. Keep going and you'll feel less ridiculous once you start getting into it.

Only one word of caution: work out an agreed "stop-now" signal before starting anything. This is particularly important if your sex games include bondage or spanking. Part of the fantasy may be the person begging for mercy, but how are you supposed to know whether it's real or feigned without a sign? Apart from that, the world is your stage and you're the superstars!

GOOD VIBRATIONS: SEX TOYS TRIED AND TESTED

Will sex aids send you to heaven or the nearest hospital? Are they a waste of time and money or a wickedly easy way to electrify your sex life? If the question is "Why use sex aids?" the answer has to be "Why not?" After all, they've been around for the last twenty-five hundred years and show no signs of disappearing! The ancient Egyptians used dildos, the Romans made candles in the shape of (rather enormous) penises, and the ancient Chinese invented the first "cock ring" by binding the base of the penis with silk. According to the erotica shops I canvassed, sex aids, particularly *female* sex toys, are selling as fast as Big Macs. While they'll never replace the real thing, say the managers, they put people in control of their own sexuality.

Today's toys are much more than playthings. The humble vibrator can be a lifeline for women who've had problems having an orgasm and many of the new aids are designed to improve vaginal muscle control. For every woman who squeals in horror at the mere mention of a sex toy, there's another who won't leave home without hers. Join the club. Don't just have a giggle at the hens' night, buy some of those strap-on dildos and balls that rattle noisily around inside. Men have more than a passing fascination with any type of sex toy and the thought of you being even remotely interested in trying one will get him *very* excited.

Rather than waste valuable dollars on an expensive aid, buy a few cheaper items to start with. A lot of the time, it's the novelty factor that appeals. If you enjoy these, then it's worth making a larger investment. Don't know where to start? Take a tip from the people who bravely volunteered (well, were bribed) to tell all about their trip to toyland . . .

STA HARD Desensitizing Spray

Cost: $11.00 (bought from a sex shop)

What is it? A spray-on potion designed to prolong his erection.

Tester: Peter, 32.

Satisfaction guaranteed? "A friend recommended it, so I thought I'd give it a try. I put a bit on the end of my penis and massaged it in but it did nothing the first time. The second time, I slathered it on and felt a weird tingling sensation but that time it did work. I stayed harder for longer. No complaints."

His rating: 7/10

Fun Tongue

Cost: $124.99 (available from Web site: www.twiceassexy.com)

What is it? A bizarre, cylindrical contraption with a tongue protruding from one end. It's designed to simulate oral sex and devotees swear it's as good as the real thing—if you can stop laughing for long enough to take it seriously. Insert lubricant into a special compartment and set the (washable) tongue on one of five settings. It licks up and down, side to side, or moves in and out.

Tester: Susie, 40.

Satisfaction guaranteed? "I saw it in the window of a sex aid shop and thought, 'I've got to have it.' I tried it on my hand and it felt sensational. The first time, I put on some crotchless knickers, dimmed the lights, and watched in a mirror, but it looked so ridiculous, I couldn't stop laughing. From then on, I closed my eyes. It's wild! It feels and licks like the real thing but it doesn't look the best. A friend of mine said he'd shoot it if he saw one lying on the side of the road."

Her rating: 9/10

Pearl Bird Vibrator

Cost: $85 (bought through mail order)

What is it? It's one of Australia's most popular vibrators with "pearls" in the shaft that rotate in dizzy circles and a clitoral stimulator that also vibrates.

Tester: Marie, 31.

Satisfaction guaranteed? "I saw a show on

vibrators on TV and thought the clitoral attachment thing would make me orgasm more often. I tried it inside and the rotating beads felt quite amazing, but although the clitoral stimulator was buzzing madly, nothing happened. Then I used it outside, pressed it against my clitoris, and *wow*! The only problem is it makes orgasm so easy, you forget how to have one any other way."
Her rating: 9/10

Jelly Ribbed Duo Balls
Cost: $8.00 (bought from a sex shop)
What is it? Soft, prickly latex-covered metal balls (the size of a golf ball), joined by a string. (Picture a kinky version of Click-Clacks that kids play with.) Inserted into the vagina they move around, supposedly making you feel sexy. Manufacturers also claim they help with muscle control.
Tester: Catherine, 23.
Satisfaction guaranteed? "They were a present and I unwrapped them in front of my mother—I almost killed the friend who gave them to me, but thought, 'Hey, give it a go.' I

slathered them with lubricant and inserted the first one, waited a bit, then put the second one in as well. A 'tampon' string hangs down to get them out again. I felt full up, like I was walking around with a big penis inside. I couldn't walk naturally and took them out after about three minutes. Boring!"

Her rating: 3/10

Love Cuffs

Cost: $19.00 (bought from a women's erotica shop)

What is it? Designed for slaves to fashion as well as light bondage, fur-trimmed cuffs ensure you'll look trendy even when strapped to the bed naked.

Testers: Simon, 24, and Linda, 29.

Her satisfaction guaranteed? "Simon had been harping on for ages about tying me up so I bought him the cuffs for his birthday. Boy, was he impressed! They are really easy to use, feel soft and comfortable, and we both found them a hell of a turn-on. It's our favorite (if only) sex toy."

His satisfaction guaranteed? "The best present I've ever had."
His 'n' her rating: 10/10

Rocket Rider
Cost: $75 (bought from a sex shop)
What is it? It's a double "dong" or dildo on a vinyl harness. The wearer penetrates herself, then uses the other dildo to penetrate her boyfriend anally or, if she's a lesbian, her girlfriend either anally or vaginally. "Ultra Harness" ($170) is a quality leather alternative for true devotees.
Testers: Nathan, 36, and Rachel, 24.
Her satisfaction guaranteed? "Nathan bought it—I hid around the corner. It didn't really appeal to me at all. He wanted to give it a go first and when he strapped it on I had to fight the urge to say 'Ride 'em cowboy!' He used one dildo on me vaginally and it felt all rubbery and pinched a bit at first. But I got quite a kick out of penetrating myself and using it anally on him because I could experience what it's like to penetrate someone."

His satisfaction guaranteed? "Rachel wasn't into it that much and I was quite disappointed. But I think she got a kick out of playing 'the man.' Used with tons of lubricant, I quite enjoyed having it up my bum. Without lubricant, it hurts like hell."

Her rating: 2/10 on her; 9/10 using it on him.

His rating: 8/10

PORNOGRAPHY: WHY IT'S WORTH ANOTHER LOOK

Alex Comfort (in the infamous sex bible *The Joy of Sex*) says pornography is "the name given to any sexual literature somebody is trying to suppress." He goes on to say that "most normal people enjoy looking at sex books and reading sex fantasies—which is why abnormal people have to spend so much time and money attempting to suppress them." I'm inclined to agree with him. I strongly believe that your standard "girlie" porn mag and video (those not involving torture, violence, or children) should be available to the public. If *you* don't like them, don't buy or rent them. But you'd be surprised how many people, women included, do.

After numerous bizarre tests, which involved wiring people's genitals to machines, scientists have officially declared that women get as turned on as men by reading or watching sexually explicit material. *Gosh,* we're amazed! The dispute has never really been that uninhibited, liberated women aren't turned on by watching or reading sexy things. It's just that we're not really into that hard-core stuff. X-rated films are often dull, repetitive, and so unbelievable, we feel like laughing, not bonking. Or they're so explicit, disturbing, and in-your-face, we feel like throwing up. But even if you have suffered through one of his flicks and vowed never to watch one again, here's some good news. Switch off your preconceptions and switch on that VCR or DVD player because pornography has finally given birth to erotica—a much subtler, softer style of erotic material, often targeted specifically at women.

If he wants to watch an X-rated video, say yes, but you pick it. Select one made by women for women (they promote it heavily on the back of the video box—try any of the Candida Royalle range) and you won't be forced to watch degrading scenes or silly performances by perfectly formed females who orgasm just by looking at an erect penis. If you really don't feel comfortable or have extreme moral objections even to this new range, at least give an R-rated film a go. Pick up an old classic (like *The Postman Always Rings Twice*) or opt for a film like *Damage, The Unbearable Lightness of Being,* or *9½ Weeks* as a compromise. For those who *do* want to use erotica and pornography as an adjunct to sex, keep the following points in mind.

Do:
- Try a few before dismissing adult films, magazines, or books totally. Take it in turns

to pick one and approve the decision with your partner. If you fancy one and they don't, watch it alone.

- Have it playing in the background. Often, they're too boring to watch all the way through, but looking up at the "good bits" can be fun.

- Have a laugh and don't take them seriously. It's not real sex and there's lots of misinformation in them (like women don't need foreplay and enjoy penetration above all else).

Don't:

- Think it means your partner's not happy with you. It's a bit of fun, a way to spice things up, that's all.

- Feel guilty for feeling turned on. It doesn't mean you're perverted, dirty, or sick; it means you're human.

- Force people to watch it if it does nothing for them or they're morally opposed. They're not a prude for not wanting to, and they're entitled to dislike it.

- Stop your partner indulging if you don't like pornography and they do. Just tell them you'd rather they watched/read it alone and kept it out of your sight. Unless it's extremely disturbing stuff (violent, a snuff film or involving children, for instance), it's his or her business, not yours.
- Rely on pornography to turn you on. If the VCR or DVD player is on every time you have sex, you're getting lazy.

THREE IN A BED: THREESOMES, SWAPPING, AND GROUP SEX

"I must be the luckiest man alive," confided my friend James, two sheets to the wind. "My wife wants us to try a threesome with another woman."

"So, are you going to?" I asked him.

"Of *course!*" he spluttered. "God, what man in his right mind would knock back the chance to sleep with two women at once?" There was a telling pause. "I mean, you'd have to be a real wimp to say no, wouldn't you . . . wouldn't

"I was nineteen and had been going out with this guy for about a month. We had terrific sex but both of us knew that was all we had. We were mucking around with a girlfriend of mine who's really into sex as well and she French-kissed me as a joke, to see if he got jealous. He pretended to, so we hammed it up a bit and somewhere along the line, stopped laughing and started getting into it. It very naturally turned into a threesome and all of us enjoyed it, but no one instigated a repeat performance. My girlfriend and I haven't mentioned it since."
Debbie, 31, receptionist

you? It's every bloke's dream . . . isn't it?"

"But not yours," I said, taking a gamble.

"No," he admitted, embarrassed as hell. "Truth is, the idea frightens the hell out of me."

James isn't alone. While just about all of us have fantasized about threesomes and group sex, taking that leap to reality is something else. James was terrified he wouldn't be able to satisfy both women, that they'd think he was hopeless, that he'd be left out, and that his wife would turn gay and leave him.

"I'm also not entirely convinced I'll be able to handle watching someone I love getting it on with another person, male or female," he confessed sadly.

I'm with him. I'm far too jealous to share, but lots of people I know have had threesomes with varying results. Generalizing outrageously, I'd say the ones that it worked for were couples who hadn't been together long and didn't really mind their partner being with someone else. They had a play, said it made great future fantasy material, but wouldn't rush to repeat it. For older, long-term couples, it was an emotional disaster. Even if they enjoyed it at the time, most said the fallout afterward was incredibly destructive. Jealousy, "broken" trust, paranoia that their partner secretly preferred the third person—three in a bed really is dicey stuff. Convinced your relationship could handle a ménage à trois? Read this first.

Why we want to do it

Often, threesomes appeal because we're too lazy to put the work in to boost a flagging sex life. We think a quicker, easier way to add spice is to introduce a third party—let them do the work. On the other hand, lots of us are aroused by the sight and sounds of others having sex—that's why we watch erotic videos. It can be instructive to watch other people's sexual techniques, it can make us feel desirable if there's more than one person enjoying our body, it undoubtedly adds variety, and, of course, it's taboo. The thrill of doing something both naughty and novel is often a turn-on in itself.

Some like the idea of being the center of attention and the thought of all that pleasure—*two* tongues, *two* sets of hands, *two* penises or vaginas—sounds great. In our fantasy, many of us cast

> "My boyfriend called his flatmate in while we were having sex. I said nothing because I knew it was what my boyfriend wanted. When his friend said he was getting a hard-on, my boyfriend asked him to join us. They had a 'sandwich': my boyfriend penetrated me anally, the other guy vaginally. They'd obviously discussed it before. I felt like a whore."
> Judith, 22, promotions manager

ourselves in the taking role. Generally, women are more aroused by the two women and a man combination than men are by two men and one woman.

Threesomes sometimes seem like a natural solution to couples who are bored with each other but don't want to leave or do something behind their back. Doing it in front of their partner seems less of a betrayal and most imagine the third person as an enjoyable addition rather than a threat. The people I interviewed indulged with like-minded friends, placed or answered an ad in the personals, or went to a massage parlor that catered to couples. Even if the experience was positive, in most cases, once was enough—they satisfied their curiosity but found one-on-one sex ultimately more fulfilling.

What can go wrong

Real life is very different from fantasy. Couples who love each other usually have a hard time seeing their partners with someone else and often the physical pleasure dulls because of the strong negative emotions threesomes bring up. Most of us are pretty territorial about relationships and our partners and not used to sharing them, so there's often jealousy (of the third person's body, technique, how your partner related to them). Three people in one bed is, by virtue of the fact that it's an uneven number, unequal—someone usually fancies someone else more and the attention seems to tilt that way.

After the thrill's worn off (and perhaps the alcohol—a few drinks can do wonders for turning us on physically and off mentally), lots of people feel guilty and resentful (particularly if they were talked into it), ashamed, "cheap," or disgusted with themselves. But the most common negative of all is feeling betrayed and that trust has disappeared. "I can't get the images out of my head" and "I'm scared they'll see them without me" were common comments from the people I surveyed. If your partner wants a repeat and you don't, you feel threatened. Sometimes wanting group sex is a sign of immaturity. It's all about instant gratification and it's far less personal than the one-on-one variety. It can also mean one or both of you have intimacy problems.

In a sense, going along to an arranged sex party is more honest and less tricky than a threesome with a friend. Everyone knows what they're there for, there's little chance of a relationship developing because people swap around a lot, and you're not likely to see each other again. "Swinging" or "swapping" usually means your partner's not in the same room or doing it in front of you so there are no nasty images to replay in your head. Groups that organize swapping parties also usually enforce set rules about using condoms and stopping if one person isn't enjoying it.

If you are going to give it a whirl

If you decide to go ahead, here's what you should do:

- Have condoms ready.
- Talk through what will happen: what's on, what isn't. Is kissing allowed? What if one person wants to stop and the other doesn't? Spell out who's having sex with whom. Seeing your boyfriend take another guy's penis into his mouth can be pretty shocking if it didn't occur to you the two men would have sex as well.
- As a couple, ask yourselves: Are we good at communicating, problem-solving, and negotiating? You need all three skills to get through this one.
- Ask yourself: *Do* I feel comfortable having three-way sex? Do I feel comfortable about *my partner* having sex with someone else? If you're not 100 percent sure of either, don't do it.
- Examine your motives. Are you trying to hang on to someone by agreeing? Do you feel forced into it? Then don't do it.
- If you're intent on spicing up your sex life with other people, would you be better off agreeing on an open relationship, making a

few rules like always using condoms, and then not talking about it? You don't have to have sex with someone new together.

Dear Diary, I had sex today and it was . . .

David
David, 21, admits he's as promiscuous as he possibly can be and uninterested in a long-term monogamous relationship right now. He manages a gym.

Week one
Last night I was out at my usual club and made instant eye contact with a girl that oozed "fuck me." I got close to her and tried to pick up if the vibes were positive or negative, though even if they're negative, I'll still go for it. She started dancing so I danced with her and without speaking a word, we started kissing. I took her out to the back of my four-wheel drive and we had sex. Immediately after it was over, I thought, "Why did I bother?" I should have jacked off—it would have been much more pleasurable. The sluts

never live up to expectations. There's no challenge. This girl left me, went back inside and I saw her leave to do the same thing with another guy within half an hour. When I say slut, I mean slut.

I went out with Diane tonight, a "nice girl" I met through some friends. We had dinner and she's pretty, though pretty stupid as well. She came back to my place and it was obvious she expected sex, which is weird. She comes from a well-to-do family and I thought she'd be different. I obliged but she freaked out because I couldn't come with a condom on. I never can. I have to almost get there, then pull out, take it off, and finish myself off with my hand. Eighty percent of girls don't mind but some react badly. They always think it's their fault. I can always get it up and going but ejaculating isn't the automatic process girls think it is. It goes back to when I was seventeen. I was with this girl and we had a wild weekend of sex and I came twenty-one times in three days. I don't know if it's psychological but since then, I've been pushing to come twice in a weekend. I remember feeling so drained and worn out afterward, I felt physically sick. It doesn't bother me though. Sex feels great even if I don't ejaculate.

Week two

Trish was at the club last night and I'm wondering if she's still a virgin. My best friend and I had a threesome with this girl a month ago. We met her at a party and had her outside, in full view of anyone who wanted to watch, but she'd only do oral sex. No penetration whatsoever. She said it was because she was a virgin and I was like, "Yeah, right," but she loved sucking penises and she swallowed every drop. (It's a big thing swallowing. The only thing that's better is if she swallows most of it but some sperm's trickling out of her mouth. That is so hot!) I didn't for a minute believe Trish but her best friend swears it's true. She really is a virgin.

I've just had the worst sex experience of my life. I went to go down on this girl and I was hit by a cloud of odor that turned my stomach. I literally dry retched. The girl must have had a yeast infection because no one could smell like that naturally. I still feel sick just thinking about it.

Week three
I watched a girl for two hours last night and she was something else. So beautiful and fresh I didn't want to have sex with her; I knew I wanted a relationship just by looking at her. I blundered my way through a conversation but she's already got a boyfriend. Bummer. Despite what I sound like, I do think it's feasible to have sex with one person for the rest of your life. You'd have to love them incredibly and she'd have to be adventurous, open to new ideas and interested in doing the things I like, but it's possible. Every guy strays but I think you'd be surprised how many stay faithful when they really love their wives or girlfriends. In one sense, I'm relieved that girl had a boyfriend. I would have fallen for her for sure.

Week four
Writing this diary has made me think about my sex life. I counted up how many women I've

slept with over the past year and didn't know whether to boast or be horrified. I go through periods where I'm picking up two to three girls a week for three to four months. Then I start feeling really dirty and think, "Slow down. You're hurting people." You bonk girls once and they want you to call them, so I usually take them out one more time. But then, they want more and say, "Didn't that mean anything to you?" How do you tell them, "No, the sex didn't and you didn't"? I don't mean to hurt them but I know I do.

My sex life is . . . Totally wild and depraved. I don't think I'll ever get sick of seeing a girl naked; I don't think men ever get over it even if they've been with the same woman for years. Single sex is better than the sex I had with a three-year live-in girlfriend. When she said no to sex, I used to feel very disheartened. I'd think, "I'm losing it. She doesn't want me" and I'd never be sure if she was doing it to wield power over me, like "I've got what you want but you can't have it." I'd love to have sex several times a day—it doesn't matter that I couldn't ejaculate most of the time. My worst nightmare would be to fall in love with some girl who only wanted missionary-style sex. I hate it. I like doing it doggie-style because that's the only chance I have of coming.

Putting Out Fires

....

Q&A QUICKIE
What do I do if I'm bored with sex?
I've been in the same relationship for
years and we've done just about
everything already. Is it inevitable
that sex dies?

Nothing gets my blood boiling more than when people say to me, "It's natural for sex to die. There's nothing you can do about it." The sort of people who feed me that drivel take great offense at my standard reply of "Actually there are lots of things you can do to keep sex hot, you just have to work at it" because they're

Take a good long look at your partner before waltzing down that wedding aisle: you could end up looking just like them! Just as pets often resemble their owners, evidence is now emerging that married couples look frighteningly similar after years together.

lazy. The only advantage new lovers have over long-term ones is newness—the thrill of conquering unknown territory. Pretty insignificant when weighed against the positives: feeling comfortable with each other, talking openly, and enjoying a total lack of inhibition because you trust each other implicitly. Believing sex always fizzles out eventually is like not applying for a job because you're convinced you won't get it. Who knows what might happen if you made the effort? It's the same with your sex life. It's *common* for couples to lose the sexual fizz but it's *preventable*. This whole book is devoted to suggesting ways to make sex varied and better. Forgive me for not believing that you've done "everything" already, but I don't.

Why do I find sex less exciting once I fall in love?

When we sleep with someone purely for sex, we can be as wanton and wicked as we like because we don't really care what they think of us. Once we decide we like them and do care, it's like a bucket of freezing water is poured over any and all sexual fantasies and desires that aren't considered "normal." Will he think I'm slutty? Will she think I'm weird? We switch from horny lover role to what we think is husband or wife material. Talk to your partner next time you feel like this, hopefully having a laugh about how silly your fears are. If they do expect you to act differently in bed now you're an item, I'd be considering whether I wanted to be.

I'm always the one to initiate sex and I hate the fact that she doesn't.

When you initiate sex, does she enthusiastically respond or seem halfhearted? If it's the first scenario, she may feel she needs permission (you suggesting it first) because good girls shouldn't really like it *that* much. Or perhaps you have a much higher libido than she does and simply want sex more often (she doesn't get a *chance* to get horny because you're always jumping in first). If she's lukewarm to your suggestions, she probably doesn't enjoy sex (with you or at all) and does it just because she has to. Ask her why. Maybe you're a bad lover and she's too shy to tell you. Ask her if there's anything you can do to make it more enjoyable. Wine and dine her, massage her, give her lots of foreplay and see if that makes a difference. If something feels good we *like* doing it often.

How come I always end up having sex his way?

I don't know. Presumably you can speak. Get a grip, girl! Tell him you want to try something new or just take control and jump on top of him. If you lie back like a receptacle, can you blame him for assuming you want him to call the shots?

My girlfriend loves sex but hates quickies. Why?

It could be something as simple as this: it takes her awhile to lubricate. Buy some lubricant and see if that helps. Lots of women get turned on rapidly mentally, but it takes awhile for their body to follow (and "dry" sex isn't fun). Ask *her* why she doesn't like them. Quickies are a great adjunct to leisurely sex, but if you opt for one every second session, I don't blame her for not being thrilled.

Who sleeps in the wet spot?

One night you do, the next he does.

How do I say no to sex without upsetting him?

Here's a novel concept: don't worry if you do. Most men would prefer you say no than have sex when you don't want to. If he does want you to perform on demand, change partners. The fact is, you don't need his permission to refuse. If you're polite and he's a nice guy, he might well roll over huffily and sulk for a while but, hopefully, he'll be aware that he's acting childishly. How best to say thanks but no thanks? That really depends on the guy. Try telling the truth. "I'm exhausted and just feel like sleep" or "I don't know why, I just don't feel like it. Let's have a cuddle instead." Make it clear that you're rejecting sex, not him, and he should handle it okay.

How do I tell a much-loved partner that he's abysmal in bed without using words?

Try using body language to get the message across. When he does something you do like, exaggerate your response: moan loudly, move closer, kiss him harder so he can't help but get the message that you like what he's doing. If you don't like something, make that abundantly clear as well: twist away, lift your body away from his touch or (better) redirect his hand, mouth, or penis. Most people do to their partners what they'd like done to them. If you like having your ear licked and bitten, you'll lick and bite his. Slip this into a conversation as a bit of interesting trivia then give him the attention *you'd* like the next time you're in bed.

If he still doesn't get the hint, you've got no other option but to talk to him. You really are better off using words than actions anyway. Just about every woman has lain there thinking, "If I just hang in there a bit longer, he's *bound* to hit the right spot sooner or later." But squirm all you want, sometimes it just isn't going to happen unless you say something. Sadly, you're not alone in wanting to stay silent. A lot of people don't say anything in bed, let alone "Let me have it harder and a little to the left." But how's he going to know that you think he's boring unless you tell him?

"I was bonking a girl doggie-style once and really getting into it, but all she could talk about was how big her bum must look. It was a turn-off! We don't notice your flaws so there's no need to hide them. When we stare at you walking around naked, we're appreciating the good bits, not focusing on what you think are the bad."
Jeremy, 18, bartender

I like doing "kinky" things but get the feeling my current lover would be horrified. How do I feel her out about this, without embarrassing myself or scaring her off?

It really depends on what you and she define as kinky. No matter how broad-minded your lover is, I wouldn't suggest striding into the bedroom, dressed in her underwear, without giving her a little warning first. But if "kinky" simply means trying something new, try using the third-person perspective to introduce a tricky topic. Say, "I heard a story about a friend who" or "I had a dream about" and see what reaction you get. Or say you've got a fantasy about such-and-such. That way, you're

"Women who can achieve that up-but-falling-down look with their hair or put on a show and parade their new underwear, you can't help but love them. The sight of her lying deliberately arranged on the bed in my underwear gives me an erection so hard, I could carve my initials in it."
Phillip, 23, photographer

insinuating rather than directly propositioning, which can be erotic anyway. If she nervously starts wringing her hands, there's your answer. If she looks interested, follow it up with "Why don't we try it next time?"

Will he think I've "been around" if I suggest something unusual?

Again, it depends on what it is, but I'd imagine most guys would be ecstatic rather than horrified if you'd like to try something new. If he thinks you're not a "nice girl" for wanting to experiment, you're probably mismatched anyway. Do you want to spend the rest of your life acting like a nun?

Often, I don't orgasm during intercourse even though my lover always does. I know I could come if he gave me oral sex afterward. Is it fair to ask?

Is it fair that he has an orgasm and you don't? Of course it's fair to expect to feel satisfied at the end of making love. Just bear in mind that men aren't as blasé about body secretions as women are (they've never had to cope with things like periods), but a quick one-minute wash in the bathroom is likely to change his mind until he loosens up a little. Alternatively, have an orgasm before intercourse through oral sex, or ask him to manually masturbate you with his fingers afterward. Better still, get him to stimulate your clitoris *during* intercourse.

If he/she gives me an orgasm through oral sex, do I have to give him/her one, too?

You probably are expected to reciprocate, but it doesn't have to be immediately. Take turns. Lots of couples plan sex sessions where one partner concentrates on the other. One day, he can massage you, finish with oral sex, and let you drift straight off into a delicious sleep; the next time, you do the same for him.

> "I always feel vulnerable after sex—I think all women do. I don't want poetry, just some sort of acknowledgment that you enjoyed it and I wasn't just a notch on the bedpost."
> Katherine, 25, chef

SEX FOR SEX'S SAKE: THE RULES

If you've just come out of a long-term relationship (and can't bear to dive into another), haven't got time for a love affair because your career is all-consuming, or have simply met someone who makes you boil down under but leaves you cold above, a lust affair could be *just* what the sex therapist ordered.

Men have been having sex affairs since God said, "Let there be light" (even if their partners didn't realize it). Now, lots of confident girls with raging libidos and a guilt-free attitude to satisfying them are also able to separate sex from love. They're not searching for Mr. Right or even a commitment for a date on Saturday night: all they want is good sex and a good time.

If that's you, go for it! But be careful, not just with your sexual health and personal safety, but with your emotional health as

Women who stay single are more likely to be among the most intelligent and highly educated of their sex, and to have reached top levels of achievement. Never-married men tend to be the exact opposite.

well. Just because there's no commitment to be monogamous doesn't mean either of you have the right to treat each other badly. If you're going to indulge, here are the rules:

- **Refuse to feel guilty.** If you suffer even the faintest twinge of guilt, sex-only affairs aren't for you. If you find you're waking up feeling depressed or bad about yourself, don't do it again. People in casual relationships are exploiting each other—which is fine as long as that's what they both want. Just remember there's a huge difference between having sex and making love. He's not going to send flowers, she's not going to call to say good night. So there's no reason to pretend you don't usually do this sort of thing, even if you don't. If he thinks you're a bit easy, who cares?
- **Use condoms every single time.** If I have to explain why, you're not a candidate.
- **Use backup contraception.** Again, for obvious reasons.
- **Do it for the right reasons.** Casual sex may make you feel sexy, attractive, and desirable

but it won't make you feel special or loved. If you're having sex just to get the hug at the end, stop kidding yourself. Lust affairs are conducted for sheer pleasure. Don't sleep with someone simply to reaffirm your attractiveness.

- **Let go of any inhibitions.** A lot of women find they're much less inhibited with a guy they don't care about. After all, does it matter if he thinks you're fat or kinky? If you've always wanted to have someone tie you up and lick cream off your body, this is your man.
- **Don't broadcast your affairs.** Some women will brand you just as readily as some men will. It's your business, not theirs.
- **Stay in control by being honest with each other.** Establish upfront that you want uncomplicated sex and not a relationship. If you feel yourself falling for them, let them know. They might feel the same. If they don't, stop seeing them and find someone else. Great sex isn't worth a broken heart.
- **Be nice to each other.** He's got a body that

makes you wet just looking at it? Tell him. She's so erotic, you're convinced she'll be in your fantasies forever? Ditto. Compliments don't equal commitment.

- **Pick your partners carefully.** If you feel like sex and don't meet someone who measures up, go home and masturbate instead. Choose partners whom you like and who make you feel good about yourself. Other people's husbands, wives, girlfriends, and boyfriends are off-limits; and don't sleep with friends of friends unless you can cope with the rumor mill.

- **If you're female, don't put yourself in risky situations.** Be super-safety conscious and trust your gut reactions. If you feel it's wrong and the guy's a bit dodgy, don't do it. It's safer to take him back to your place (with a flatmate home and in the next room) than it is to go back to his. If you've seen him a few times and trust him enough to go to his place, leave his address and phone number with someone *you* trust.

SEX ON HOLIDAY

The sun's shining, the waves are lapping, and the hardest decision you've had to make all week is which way to point your deck chair. That wonderfully relaxed holiday mood can make it seem like the yukkies of life don't exist. Unfortunately AIDS, STDs, and unwanted pregnancies don't disappear just because you're feeling blissfully brain-dead. Holidays are danger time for many people. Make sure *you* don't come home with more souvenirs than you'd bargained on.

- Pack condoms, lubricant, and enough supplies of your chosen contraceptive to last the trip, plus spares. (It's tough enough asking for directions when you can't speak the language; try explaining what a flat-spring diaphragm is and why you need one *now*!)

- Don't rely on the calendar, mucus, or withdrawal methods. Symptothermal methods are notoriously unreliable at the best of times, worse on holidays. Time differences and long flights play havoc with your menstrual cycle and it's difficult to keep track of fertile days. Heat, lounging around in spas, a case of thrush brought on by preholiday panic, all can affect vaginal secretions. Use condoms and lubricant instead; they'll protect you against pregnancy, HIV, and STDs. Don't use the withdrawal method with holiday romancers. It's easy enough for a boyfriend to get carried away—can you trust a stranger to keep his word?

- It's Tuesday there and Thursday in Australia, so when should you take the Pill? Keep your watch on "home" time during the flight and take the tablets as usual. When you get to your destination, take a tablet in the morning or evening (whichever is usual for you), even if it means taking it early. Then take one tablet per day until the flight home. Keep your watch on "holiday" time on the flight back and continue taking

> "He was the first guy I'd ever slept with, a doctor, and twelve years older than me. He gave me hepatitis and I was sick for months. I learned the hard way why condoms are a must."
> Flavia, 22, waitress

the tablets. When you get home, repeat the process: take a tablet that morning or evening, then settle back into your old routine. Remember that the Pill's effectiveness is hampered by holiday bugs that cause vomiting and diarrhea. If you vomit within an hour of taking it, it's not been absorbed. Use condoms or a diaphragm as backup.

- If you use a diaphragm, pack two and keep them in separate bags (in case you lose a suitcase). Flying, swimming in saltwater, even scuba diving won't affect your diaphragm. Just remember it must stay in for six hours, so don't get confused with changing time zones. If you get a particularly bad bout of gastric illness (or anything else that causes you to drop eleven pounds or more), your diaphragm may be the wrong size and ineffective. That new, flat tummy won't stay flat for long if you're pregnant!

- Practice safe sex in all senses. What might pass as flirting back home may be interpreted as a blatant invitation for sex somewhere else. Quiz your travel agent on the customs and morals of the country you're visiting. And don't assume any guy you invite in for coffee will behave like a gentleman— no matter what country you're in.

Dear Diary, I had sex today and it was . . .

Stephen

Stephen, 28, has been married for two years. He's a stockbroker and says he loves his wife more now than when they first got married.

Week one

I arrive home from a fourteen-hour workday and Jess is in a mad panic, running around with her underwear on because she's late meeting a girlfriend. I try to talk her into a quickie because she looks so sexy but no way. She won't even laugh with me. I get out a porn video (Jess hates them) and masturbate instead. When she comes home, she's tipsy and sits on my lap and gives me a deep kiss, using her tongue. Ironically, now it's me who can't be bothered. The day's caught up with me.

The next morning I wake up "pee-proud" (my grandmother's term for a morning erection). I wake Jess by stroking and licking her back but she's hungover and not interested. I try really hard not to act pissed off but she knows I am and gets shitty herself. Somehow, this turns into a huge row and ruins the weekend.

Week two

The three-day war is over and Jess finally lets me have sex with her. She's really wet and I have to think about football to stop orgasming within a second. It's funny, even though she's really lubricated I get the feeling she's not really into it. Afterward, we watch the soaps and she's asleep within two minutes. I guess she was tired.

Jess's best friend has the best body I've ever seen in the flesh. She knows it and always wears the shortest skirts. Tanya was bending over at a lunch and she's got the most fabulous legs: no lumpy bits, just smooth flesh. Jess caught me watching, leaned over, and felt to see if I had an erection. It was certainly getting there. She was not impressed and announced to the whole table what had happened. I laughed it off but was totally pissed off. We had a huge row when we got home, so—no sex *again*.

Week three
Jess's sexual calendar is so predictable, I could literally circle the days when she'll feel like it and when she won't. The week before her period she turns into this intense nympho and screws really seriously, closes her eyes and concentrates like this is the last time ever. Jess also likes sex during her period and I have to pretend I do, too. Actually, I hate it, but Jess is a real feminist and if I dared to admit I'm turned off by menstrual blood I'd never hear the end of it.

My boss just got a new secretary. She flirted with me today and asked me to go to lunch. I said fine, I like having women as friends, but made it very clear I was married and very happily so. Her behavior changed after that—she wasn't interested in getting to know me as a person, just a potential Mr. Right. Stupid woman. It really annoyed me.

Week four

I'm raring to go and so is Jess—a rare moment in our household. She pulls on this amazing two-piece underwear thing, all white and virginal, which she knows I love. She gives me a massage and I'm so tense and it feels so good, I almost lose the urge and just want to sleep. But then her tongue flicks over my penis and it responds, though not as quick as my brain does, so I move down on her. I love giving Jess oral sex. I love the smell of her. If I could bottle her vaginal juices I would. Sometimes, if she's really turned on and climaxes loudly, I'll almost come without any stimulation of my genitals at all. This session is so good, I feel really vulnerable afterward. I bury my nose in her hair and pray to God she'll never leave me.

My sex life is . . . Up and down but satisfying. I guess it reflects our relationship. We argue a lot, which stops us from having sex as often as I'd like but that's okay; I like Jess's spirit and married a passionate woman. I have no desire for sex with anyone else. Jess turns me on as much now as she did when I first met her and I don't see why her appeal will ever wear off. We're experimenting more now and she's not backward in coming forward about her desires. I think I scored lucky!

7

PS: Don't Get Burned!

·····································

Like most diseases, STDs (sexually transmitted diseases) aren't fussy and you can't pick the people who have one. Avoid "dirty," "promiscuous," or "bad boy/wild girl" types all you like, but if you think you're safe having sex only with "sweet," "nice," "clean," or "innocent" people, you're being unbelievably naive. Ditto those who skip the condoms because they have asked their partner if they have any symptoms. Let's face it, they're hardly going to remove their hands from your breasts, sit back, and say, "Well, now that you mention it, I had these godawful blisters on my penis yesterday and now they've turned into pus-infected ulcers." Besides, they may not have noticed anything unusual because some STDs are alarmingly symptom-free.

Sex can give us the most pleasurable moments of our life—and the most painful. Falling pregnant by the waiter in Greece who did more than just lay the table or discovering a T-shirt wasn't the only thing your ex left behind are both very real consequences of not treating sex with the respect it demands. Don't kid yourself: having sex can be a dangerous business. Protect your heart by using common sense, protect your parts by using condoms, and protect against pregnancy by using reliable contraceptives. At the risk of sounding like your mother, pulling on that condom will not only save you heartache, it could save your life.

HOW TO USE A CONDOM

1. Be careful when you're unwrapping it. Don't rip the packet open with abandon (and don't even think about doing it with your teeth). Rings and fingernails can snag,

and while condoms are tough, they're not *that* tough.

2. Wait until he's erect. Put the condom on *before* the penis touches the vagina but only when he's hard.

3. Leave the condom unrolled and squeeze the tip to get rid of any air. Hold it against the tip of the penis, then . . .

4. Gently unroll the condom, all the way down to the base of the penis. Smooth out any air bubbles once it's on. Apply some extra *water-based* lubricant on the outside of the condom even if it's been prelubricated.

5. Have fun—guilt-free!

6. Withdraw the penis *immediately* after ejaculation while it's still erect. One of you should hold the condom firmly at the base of the penis while he withdraws, to stop it from slipping off or any sperm from leaking out.

7. Point the penis downward and slip the condom off carefully.

8. Remember you can only use a condom once. If you want to have sex again, get him to wash his penis and use a new one.

9. Tie a knot in the used condom, wrap it in paper, and put it in a bin. Don't flush it down the loo—it's not biodegradeable. Do you enjoy dragging used condoms along with your toes while walking on your local beach?

10. Score full marks for putting it on with your mouth. If you can cope with the taste, unwrap it and place it (unrolled) on the top of your tongue, the open end facing upward. The first time, cheat and use your fingers to position it over the penis head, then use your tongue and mouth to unroll it.

HOT SEX:
HOW TO DO IT

Tracey Cox

"A hilarious read with the power to transform your sex life from average to outstanding overnight." *FHM* magazine

Practical, down-to-earth, explicit, and fun, HOT SEX is the must-have sex and relationships book for every woman and man.

It's the perfect bedtime reading for two, an easy-to-follow guide that cuts straight to the nitty-gritty to deliver candid advice with a healthy dose of humor. Packed with tips and techniques that work, HOT SEX includes everything from a blow-by-blow, step-by-step guide to oral sex to finding (and figuring out) your G-spot.

Whether you're a beginner or an old hand, get into HOT SEX—the only how-to that really tells you how to do it!

BANTAM BOOKS

HOT RELATIONSHIPS:
HOW TO HAVE ONE

Tracey Cox

Are you madly in love or driven mad by it? Happily single or looking for a partner? Living together, married with kids, or dumped and desperate? Whatever the state of your love life, HOT RELATIONSHIPS has the answers to all your dating and relating dilemmas.

Funny, practical, and refreshingly realistic, it's packed with advice on everything from flirting and flings to monogamy and marriage. There's hot tips on getting over an ex, where to meet a partner, how to spot the losers, and how to breeze through that first date, as well as hints on fixing the fights, surviving jealousy and infidelity, and breaking bad love habits.

A must-have manual for singles, couples, men, and women, HOT RELATIONSHIPS shows you how to have one—and how to keep it that way.

BANTAM BOOKS

Tracey Cox is an international sex and relationships counselor, writer, and TV presenter. Her first book, *Hot Sex: How to Do It*, became an instant best seller worldwide. Flirty, frank, and funny, it's now on sale in more than 120 countries—and has turned her into a celebrity "sexpert." Tracey's second book, *Hot Relationships: How to Have One*, was also a runaway success and is available in more than thirty countries. It has firmly established her as an influential teacher of relationship skills, including body language. If you've got questions or problems with your sex life or love life, chances are she's got the answers!

In between writing and promoting her books, Tracey starred in several television shows in the UK, including the BBC series *Would Like to Meet*. She is also featured on the US version of that show, *Date Patrol*. A former associate editor of Australian *Cosmopolitan*, Tracey has also written for most major women's magazines internationally. She is consistently interviewed and quoted in magazines and newspapers worldwide as a sex and relationships expert. Her Web site is www.traceycox.com.